Interface between Regulation and Statistics in Drug Development

Chapman & Hall/CRC Biostatistics Series

Recently Published Titles

Geospatial Health Data: Modeling and Visualization with R-INLA and Shiny
Paula Moraga

Artificial Intelligence for Drug Development, Precision Medicine, and Healthcare
Mark Chang

Bayesian Methods in Pharmaceutical Research
Emmanuel Lesaffre, Gianluca Baio, Bruno Boulanger

Biomarker Analysis in Clinical Trials with R
Nusrat Rabbee

Interface between Regulation and Statistics in Drug Development
Demissie Alemayehu, Birol Emir, Michael Gaffney

Medical Risk Prediction Models: With Ties to Machine
LearningThomas A Gerds, Michael W. Kattan

Real-World Evidence in Drug Development and Evaluation
Harry Yang, Binbing Yu

For more information about this series, please visit:
https://www.routledge.com/Chapman--Hall-CRC-Biostatistics-Series/book-series/CHBIOSTATIS

Interface between Regulation and Statistics in Drug Development

Demissie Alemayehu
Birol Emir
Michael Gaffney

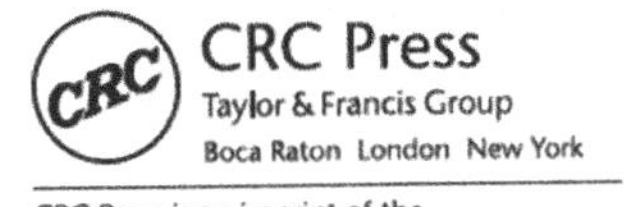

CRC Press is an imprint of the
Taylor & Francis Group, an informa business

First edition published 2021
by CRC Press
6000 Broken Sound Parkway NW, Suite 300, Boca Raton, FL 33487-2742

and by CRC Press
2 Park Square, Milton Park, Abingdon, Oxon OX14 4RN

Library of Congress Cataloging-in-Publication Data
Names: Alemayehu, Demissie, editor. | Emir, Birol, editor. | Gaffney, Michael, active 1983, editor.
Title: Interface between regulation and statistics in drug development / edited by
Demissie Alemayehu, Birol Emir, Michael Gaffney. Description: First edition. |
Boca Raton: CRC Press, 2021. | Includes bibliographical references and index.
Identifiers: LCCN 2020025306 (print) | LCCN 2020025307 (ebook) |
ISBN 9780367490485 (hardback) | ISBN 9780367608286 (paperback) | ISBN 9781003044208 (ebook)
Subjects: LCSH: United States. Food and Drug Administration–Rules and practice. |
Drugs–United States–Testing–Statistical methods. |Drugs–Testing–Law and legislation–United States. |
Clinical trials–United States–Statistical methods. | Clinical trials–Law and legislation–United States.|
Clinical trials–Reporting–United States.| Drug development–United States. |
Pharmaceutical policy–UnitedStates. Classification: LCC RM301.27 .I58 2021 (print) |
LCC RM301.27 (ebook) |DDC 615.1072/4–dc23
LC record available at https://lccn.loc.gov/2020025306
LC ebook record available at https://lccn.loc.gov/2020025307

ISBN: 9780367490485 (hbk)
ISBN: 9781003044208 (ebk)

Typeset in Minion
by Newgen Publishing UK

Contents

Figures

Abbreviations

AC	Advisory Committee
ADDIS	Aggregate Data Drug Information System
AE	Adverse experience or event
AI	Artificial intelligence
ANCOVA	Analysis of covariance
ANOVA	Analysis of variance
AUC	Area under the curve
BCOF	Best observation or baseline observation carried-forward
BD	Briefing Document
BRAT	Benefit–Risk Action Team
BRF	Benefit–Risk Framework
CART	Classification and regression trees
CDF	Cumulative distribution function
CHMP/SAWP	Committee for Medicinal Products for Human Use/Scientific Advice Working Party
CIRS	Centre for Innovation in Regulatory Science
COA	Clinical outcome assessment
CP	Conditional power
CRM	Continual Reassessment Method
DCC	Data coordinating center
DLT	Dose Limiting Toxicity
DMC	Data Monitoring Committee
EHR	Electronic health record
EM	Expectation-maximization
EMA	European Medicines Agency
EU	European Union
FCS	Fully conditional specification

FDA	Food and Drug Administration
FDR	False discovery rate
GEE	Generalized estimating equations
GLMM	Generalized linear mixed models
HR	Hazard ratio
HRQOL	Health-related quality of life
HTA	Health technology assessment
ICH	International Conference on Harmonization
IPTW	Inverse probability of treatment weighting
IRT	Item-response theory
ITT	Intent-to-treat
IV	Instrumental variable
LASSO	Least absolute shrinkage and selection operator
LCB	Lower confidence bound
LOCF	Last observation carried-forward
LST	Large simple trial
MAR	Missing at random
MCAR	Missing completely at random
MCDA	Multiple-criteria decision analysis
MCMC	Markov chain Monte Carlo
ML	Maximum Likelihood
MMRM	Mixed-effect models for repeated measures
MNAR	Missing not at random
MTD	Maximum Tolerated Dose
NDA	New Drug Application
NDC	National Drug Code
NI	Non-interventional
NIH	National Institutes of Health
NIM	Non-inferiority Margin
NNH	Number needed to harm
NNT	Number needed to treat
NRC	National Research Council
NSAID	Nonsteroidal anti-inflammatory drug
ORR	Overall response rate
pFDR	Positive false discovery rate
PK	Pharmacokinetic
PMS	Post-Marketing Surveillance
PRO	Patient-reported outcome

PS	Propensity score
PTSD	Post-Traumatic Stress Disorder
RCT	Randomized controlled trial
REA	Relative effectiveness assessment
RP2D	Recommended Phase II dose
RWD	Real-world data
RWE	Real-world evidence
SAP	Statistical Analysis Plan
SEM	Standard error of measurements
SMAA	Stochastic multicriteria acceptability analysis
SOC	Standard of care
UMBRA	Universal Methodologies for Benefit–Risk Assessment
WOCF	Worst observation carried-forward

Authors' Disclosure

Demissie Alemayehu, Birol Emir, and Michael Gaffney are employees of Pfizer Inc. This book was prepared by the authors in their personal capacity. Views and opinions expressed in this book are those of the authors and do not necessarily reflect those of Pfizer Inc.

Acknowledgment

THE AUTHORS ARE GRATEFUL to external reviewers and Pfizer colleagues for providing constructive comments at various stages in the writing of this document. The authors are especially indebted to Jack Mardekian for his invaluable contributions in the initial planning of the book project.

Preface

THIS BOOK IS AIMED at researchers in the pharmaceutical industry and in academia with interest in drug development and, hence, in the design, conduct, analysis, and reporting of clinical trials or observational studies intended for regulatory purposes. As the title suggests, the primary focus of the book is on the intersection of statistics and regulatory affairs in the context of drug development. While the monograph is intended to be of primary interest to medical researchers and regulatory personnel, it may also serve as a useful reference for graduate students in the health sciences who wish to get an understanding of the statistical and regulatory issues that commonly arise in the course of drug development. The material is mostly written at a level that is accessible to readers with an intermediate knowledge of statistics.

The book consists of stand-alone chapters and sections, with each section dedicated to a specific topic in regulatory affairs and statistics. In each case, the authors have made a conscious effort to provide a survey of the relevant literature and to highlight emerging and current trends and guidelines for best practices, when the latter were available.

Chapter 1 highlights basic statistical and regulatory issues that must be addressed in the design, analysis, and reporting of clinical trials. In particular, due attention is paid to the role of regulations and guidance documents, and the anticipated regulatory and statistical interactions throughout the drug development continuum. Reference is also made to the evolving role of the statistician, having increasing impact and visibility, in relation to the changing regulatory and healthcare landscapes. It is also underscored that the prevailing emphasis on Big Data, modern analytics, and precision medicine will continue to present interesting challenges and opportunities both to regulatory scientists and statisticians.

The primary purpose of Chapter 2 is to provide a thorough discussion of major statistical issues that commonly arise in the course of drug development and regulatory interactions. The section on multiplicity outlines measures that should be taken to ensure the validity of inferential results that are intended to be the basis for regulatory decision-making. In a separate section, a thorough review of best practices is provided to handle missing values, which are ubiquitous in clinical trials, with special reference to pertinent guidelines and the emergent topic of estimands. While superiority trials are common to support drug approval, there are situations where it is essential to conduct non-inferiority studies. The regulatory requirements and underlying principles of such trials are summarized, and suggestions are provided relating to the salient points to be considered for both efficacy and safety assessment. In light of the increasing focus to accelerate drug development with speed and efficiency, a summary of a few commonly used novel approaches is provided, including adaptive and flexible designs, enrichment studies, and studies conducted under the so-called master protocols. Other topics of regulatory and statistical import covered in Chapter 2 include Bayesian approaches, issues with subgroup analysis, and the assessment of benefits and risks of pharmaceutical products.

Chapter 3 highlights the role of the statistician in the course of drug development, with especial emphasis on the skills required to ensure effective interactions with regulatory and other external bodies. In addition to the traditional tasks they perform in the design, analysis, and reporting of trials, statisticians now have an important seat in strategic decision-making, including advisory committee meetings assembled by regulatory bodies, evaluation of interim data by safety monitoring groups, and portfolio prioritization discussions by pharmaceutical executives.

Finally, the focus of Chapter 4 is mainly on trending topics in drug development, with emphasis on the current regulatory thinking and the associated challenges and opportunities. Although the experiences of pharmaceutical companies and regulatory bodies with some of the topics may be limited, there is a growing interest in embedding them in the current drug development paradigm. Notable examples include the role of patient-reported outcomes and their use in fostering patient-centric drug development, and the implication of the digital revolution toward advancing personalized medicine.

While it is recognized that the various topics covered in our book may be available in the literature, including guidance documents issued by the US Food and Drug Administration and other regulatory agencies, to our knowledge, there is no comparable source that provides a coherent overview of the issues addressed in this book. It is, therefore, hoped that the book will serve an essential purpose, presenting a lucid exposition of the interplay between regulatory science and statistics, and thereby contributing to the achievement of the overarching goal of bringing new medicines to patients that need them.

D.A., B.E., & M.G., Authors

About the Authors

Demissie Alemayehu, PhD, is Vice President and Head of the Statistical Research and Data Science Center at Pfizer Inc. He is a Fellow of the American Statistical Association, has published widely, and has served on the editorial boards of major journals, including the *Journal of the American Statistical Association* and the *Journal of Nonparametric Statistics*. Additionally, he has been on the faculties of both Columbia University and Western Michigan University. He has co-authored a monograph entitled *Patient-Reported Outcomes: Measurement, Implementation and Interpretation* and co-edited another, *Statistical Topics in Health Economics and Outcome Research*, both published by Chapman & Hall/CRC Press.

Birol Emir, PhD, is Senior Director and Statistics Lead of Real-World Evidence (RWE) at Pfizer Inc. In addition, Dr. Emir has been serving as Adjunct Professor of Statistics and Lecturer at Columbia University in New York and as an External PhD Committee Member at Graduate School of Arts and Sciences, Rutgers, the State University of New Jersey. Recently, his primary focuses have been on Big Data, predictive modeling, and genomic data analysis. He has numerous publications in refereed journals, and he has co-edited *Statistical Topics in Health Economics and Outcome Research*, published by Chapman & Hall/CRC Press. He has taught many short courses and has given several invited presentations.

Michael Gaffney, PhD, is Vice President of Statistics at Pfizer, and earned his PhD from New York University School of Environmental Medicine with his dissertation in the area of multistage model of cancer induction. Dr. Gaffney has spent his 46-year career in pharmaceutical research concentrating in the areas of design and analysis of clinical trials and regulatory interaction for drug approval and product defense. He has interacted with FDA, EMA, MHRA, and regulators in Canada and Japan on over 25 distinct regulatory approvals and product issues in many therapeutic areas. Dr. Gaffney has published 40 peer-reviewed articles and has presented at numerous scientific meetings in diverse areas of modeling cancer induction, variance components, harmonic regression, factor analysis, propensity scores, meta-analysis, large safety trials, and sample size reestimation. Dr. Gaffney was recently a member of the Council for International Organizations of Medical Sciences (CIOMS) X committee and was a co-author of *CIOMS X: Evidence Synthesis and Meta-Analysis for Drug Safety*.

CHAPTER 1

Fundamental Principles of Clinical Trials

1.1 INTRODUCTION

As a highly regulated industry, biomedical research must meet strict requirements that are encapsulated in the form of regulations, guidelines, and best practices. The principles underlying these requirements are principles of good science in general and concern the advancement of public health through state-of-the-science research, while safeguarding the rights and safety of study participants. In this section, we provide an overview of the statistical principles underpinning clinical trials intended for registration. Relevant literature on other aspects of medical research, including protection of trial subjects, investigator and sponsor responsibilities, quality assurance, and other operational requirements may be found elsewhere (see, e.g., International Conference of Harmonization 1996; World Health Organization 2002). Although clinical trials are typically classified into phases I to IV, differing mainly in scope, objective, and methodology, they all share certain fundamental principles in terms of prespecification of relevant aspects of the trial in a protocol or Statistical Analysis Plan (SAP), data processing and analytical approaches, subject safety protection, and other operational procedures. Further, they all require the institution of quality assurance processes to guarantee the integrity of the trial and the accompanying results. It is also a requirement that results of phases I–IV trials be appropriately summarized and interpreted in a study report, highlighting the strengths and weaknesses of the trial findings, and their contributions to advance medical science and public health.

Phase I trials are primarily concerned with the assessment of the safety, tolerability, and pharmacokinetic (PK) profiles of the investigational agent using healthy volunteers. PK studies are especially conducted to assess how a drug is absorbed, distributed, metabolized, and excreted in a human body. In general, a key objective of Phase I research is the identification of the optimal doses for use in subsequent Phase II studies. The determination of a Maximum Tolerated Dose (MTD) with acceptable Dose Limiting Toxicity (DLT) is typically achieved using either a rule-based or a model-based design. An example of the former is the conventional 3 + 3 cohort expansion design, in which dose escalation or de-escalation decision is made with reference to the toxicity observed on the current group of three study participants assigned to a dose. Specifically, the dose is lowered if the current dose is considered toxic; otherwise, the current dose is maintained or escalated to the next level. On the other hand, a model-based approach, such as the Continual Reassessment Method (CRM), involves fitting a dose-toxicity curve to estimate the MTD. Estimation of parameters associated with the curve may be performed either via the Maximum Likelihood (ML) or Bayesian framework. Although Phase I trials are relatively less complex than other phases, they can still pose certain operational and analytical challenges. Further, while the primary ethical consideration is to ensure that participants are not exposed to unsafe levels of the study drug, this assessment still involves a difficult benefit–risk judgment. For example, in trials involving cancer immunotherapy, the traditional Phase I paradigms appear to be challenged, especially with respect to determination of patient eligibility, as well as the MTD and PK profiles of the drug (Postel-Vinay et al. 2016).

In contrast, Phase II trials are typically conducted in a sample of the target patient population and aim at establishing preliminary evidence of efficacy and safety, and, in some cases, the optimal dose ranges. Phase II trials are often planned as two subphases (Phase IIA and IIB), depending on the complexity of the objectives and disease area. For efficiency reasons, Phase IIA trials may employ a single arm and a historical control group. This approach, while attractive, requires care to ensure minimization of bias associated with confounding factors and heterogeneity (Lara and Redman 2012). Phase IIB trials are intended to provide more definitive evidence to inform decisions to proceed into Phase III. As a result, a Phase IIB trial usually involves randomization and multiple arms, with a suitable control group. In oncology, Phase II trials are customarily conducted using flexible, multistage designs, with prespecified minimax criteria (Kramar et al. 1996). Notably, while in a typical optimal two-stage design the goal is to minimize the expected sample size under the null hypothesis, a minimax design targets minimization of the maximum sample size.

Phase III trials, generally conducted using randomized, double-blind designs, are intended to provide relatively more definitive results relating to the short- and long-term safety and efficacy of the drug under investigation. Phase III trials are often referred to as confirmatory trials and are the critical trials in the regulatory approval process. Accordingly, these studies tend to be larger than the corresponding Phase I or II trials, and may pose additional operational and analytical complexities, depending on the number of participating sites, nature of study endpoints, and study procedures. When they are conducted in multiple centers, the trials require well-established processes to ensure consistency of study conduct across the various sites. In particular, to ascertain the interpretability of data pooled from the various centers, certain measures may need to be put in place, including periodic training of site personnel and establishment of committees charged with providing guidance for data collection, study endpoint evaluation, or other aspects of the conduct of the study.

With the ever-rising cost of drug development, prolonged development time, and dwindling number of new medicines achieving marketing authorization, there has been increased focus on novel approaches to clinical development and trial design. This has particularly been the centerpiece of the Food and Drug Administration's (FDA) Critical Path Initiative, launched with the aim of improving efficiency and reducing attrition rates. Proposed approaches under that framework include use of historical data, modeling and simulation, and trial designs, such as the seamless Phase II/III trials, having greater degrees of flexibility than those employed traditionally. Although these novel approaches have tremendous potential to generate reliable information in a speedy manner, their implementation may require substantial quantitative work and operational efforts. Consequently, while there are cases of successful applications, routine use of the approaches has not yet been fully realized. In the traditional paradigm, the efficacy of the drug in the targeted population along with the manner in which it can be safely administered should be established at the end of Phase III. The drug developer then submits the entire body of research in a New Drug Application (NDA) to the regulatory agencies.

After a drug is approved and marketed, Phase IV trials are conducted to gather additional data on safety or to understand further the therapeutic value or alternative treatment strategies of the drug. In some instances, postmarketing studies may be conducted for a new indication or label enhancement. To achieve such objectives, which may also include claims about a new dosage or strength of the drug, or the way the drug is manufactured, the drug developer may file the so-called supplemental new drug application or sNDA.

When the goal is to obtain data about a drug's effectiveness, as used in the real world, or to evaluate resource utilization, non-interventional (NI) studies are carried out in a naturalistic setting. In such studies the drug is typically prescribed in accordance with the approved label, and the healthcare providers perform only procedures required in routine practice. Thus, the effectiveness of a drug evaluated through NI studies can complement the efficacy and safety data gathered in the restricted randomized controlled trials (RCTs) conducted for preapproval review by regulatory bodies. Other options include Phase IV studies that are intended for Post-Marketing Surveillance (PMS) purposes, per regulatory requirement, and disease registries, which involve patients with common characteristics and collect ongoing data over time on selected outcomes of interest. These prospective observational studies can provide valuable data on various aspects of the drug, including safety and effectiveness, but require caution in the interpretation of the results. A major drawback of such studies is the potential for bias emanating from lack of randomization. In certain situations, large simple trials (LSTs) or pragmatic trials may be conducted as a hybrid between an RCT and NI study (Maclure 2009; Patsopoulos 2011; Roehr 2013; Mentz 2016).

When it is desired to enhance administrative efficiency or minimize investigator bias, cluster randomization trials, in which the randomization unit is not the individual subject, but groups defined by suitable criteria, e.g., clinics or communities, have been proposed as a viable option (Donner and Klar 2004). From a statistical perspective, a major drawback of such studies is the loss in statistical precision relative to the corresponding RCT with the same number of subjects. Further, the analysis of data from such studies requires caution, since the techniques will need to take into account the intracluster correlation.

To ensure that the safety of study participants is protected and that the trial achieves the desired outcome, the sponsor should seek input from all applicable stakeholders, including patient advocates, key opinion leaders, and drug regulatory bodies. In addition, reference should be made to relevant guidance documents issued by regulatory agencies, especially when considering nontraditional trial designs or novel analytical approaches. In certain situations, it may also be essential to establish Data Monitoring Committees (DMCs) with a mandate to periodically assess the safety and scientific validity and integrity of clinical trials, or to make appropriate recommendations for changes in trial design or duration (Ellenberg et al. 2002; US FDA 2006).

In the rest of this chapter, we highlight some of the general statistical considerations that should be taken into account in the design, analysis, and reporting of clinical trials. In subsequent chapters, detailed descriptions of key statistical concepts will be provided, with particular reference to their importance in regulatory review and approval.

1.2 GENERAL STATISTICAL CONSIDERATIONS

1.2.1 Statistical Analysis Plan

Along with the study protocol, the Statistical Analysis Plan (SAP) is an important document that serves a useful purpose to ensure the transparency and integrity of the design, analysis, and reporting of a clinical trial. While it is expected that every protocol will consist of a statistical methodology section (see, e.g., International Conference for Harmonization of Technical Requirements for Pharmaceuticals for Human Use [ICH] E9 1998), it is customary to document detailed aspects of the analytical approaches and the basis for interpreting the study outcome in a separate SAP.

At a minimum, the SAP should include a detailed description of the following elements: trial design, randomization, sample size determination, null hypothesis, primary and secondary endpoints, decision rules for final and any interim analyses, analysis populations, analysis methods, handling of multiplicity and missing values, and details of any additional analyses not specified in the study protocol (see, e.g., Gamble et al. 2017). To the extent possible, the SAP should be consistent with the study protocol, and any deviation from the protocol should be clearly stated and justified. It is also essential to finalize the SAP as early as possible, but no later than the time when clean and validated data are available for analyses.

With the growing emphasis on the transparency of the conduct and reporting of clinical trials, it may also be advisable, under certain circumstances, to make the SAP publicly available (Finfer and Bellomo

2009). Notably, the US National Institutes of Health Final Rule for Clinical Trials Registration and Results Information Submission (2016) specifically states the conditions under which the SAP may need to be posted. National Institutes of Health, Department of Health and Human Services. Final rule for clinical trials registration and results information submission: 42 CFR Part 11. https://www.federalregister.gov/documents/2016/09/21/2016-22129/clinical-trials-registration-and-results-information-submission. Published September 21, 2016. Accessed August 10, 2029.

1.2.2 Trial Design

The success of a clinical trial to provide reliable data for decision-making is heavily dependent on the choice of a design framework that is appropriate for the trial objectives, study population, operational feasibility, and the phase of the drug development cycle. For example, crossover designs are often desired in certain early-phase trials, especially in comparative bioavailability and bioequivalence studies. While the main appeal of such designs is in the fact that each patient acts as his or her own control, their use may be limited to situations in which outcome measures can be observed in a short period of time, and where carryover effects may be minimal or could be managed by introducing a washout period. In later phases, the parallel group design is common, which invariably requires randomization, *a priori* specification of the meaningful difference between treatments, adequate statistical power to detect that difference, and institution of measures to minimize any potential bias.

Novel study designs are now available to enhance the efficiency and productivity of clinical trials. Adaptive designs permit modifications to various attributes of the trial based on analysis of data from subjects in the study, while ensuring the integrity of the trial is not compromised. The modification may involve study procedures, including eligibility criteria, dose levels, duration of treatment, or statistical techniques. Some of the commonly used adaptive design methods include adaptive randomization, group sequential designs, sample size reestimation, adaptive dose-finding designs, as well as biomarker-adaptive seamless Phase II/III trial designs (Chow et al. 2005). An important requirement in the implementation of these designs is the need to prespecify all the intended modifications and adaptations that will take place after the trial is initiated (see, e.g., FDA 2010 and EMA 2006). The areas where there is a critical need for novel design approaches include rare disease and oncology drug development. In oncology, for example, the so-called platform, basket, and umbrella studies as well as adaptive enrichment design strategies seem to be gaining increasing acceptance in recent times (Berry 2015). Such trials are intended to enhance efficiency, since they allow the investigation of many combinations of drugs and targets simultaneously (Renfro and Sargent 2017). A detailed review of commonly used enhanced clinical trial designs will be provided in Chapter 2.

1.2.3 Randomization and Blinding

When implemented appropriately, randomization ensures protection against bias associated with systematic differences between treatment groups, generally arising from imbalances in confounding factors. It also permits application of formal statistical inference techniques to rule out treatment differences that are due to the play of chance. A common randomization approach is the so-called fixed randomization, in which treatment assignment is based on sequences determined before the start of the trial. Fixed randomization may be simple or stratified (or blocked). While stratification may appear appealing in terms of ensuring balance, the operational burden may make the benefits less attractive relative to simple randomization (Schultz and Grimes 2002). In other situations, randomization may also be performed adaptively, adjusting for any imbalances in the course of the trial, using predefined prognostic factors (an approach sometimes called minimization). When practically feasible, blinding of the researchers and study subjects may be important to minimize the impact of bias associated with the expectations of study participants as well as investigators. Blinding could also improve compliance and enhance patient engagement (Schultz and Grimes 2002). As reported in Boutron et al. (2006), inadequate blinding could result in substantially large treatment effects. It is therefore essential to ensure that the blinding method is reliable, including, when possible, use of treatments identical in appearances or mode of administration.

The procedure used for randomization, and the blinding techniques should be explicitly stated in the study protocol and in subsequent reports to help regulators and readers evaluate the adequacy of the measures taken to minimize bias. In addition, there should be a clear statement of the process for breaking blind, if applicable, and the accessibility of the treatment assignment information to various stakeholders associated with the trial.

1.2.4 Statistical Methodology

The statistical methods intended for the analysis of the primary and secondary endpoints are expected to be specified in the study protocol or SAP and executed as planned. In choosing a model for the primary or secondary analysis, several factors should be taken into account. First, the model should be in consonance with the study design, randomization scheme, and the known properties of the outcome variables. In addition, one should consider the need for the inclusion of any covariates in the model; and, if so, how to handle interactions. Further, sufficient details should be provided up front about the imputation of missing values, especially when there are repeated measurements on the outcome variable, and any adjustment that may be needed to address multiplicity issues, if applicable.

In practice, there may be deviations from the assumptions underlying the prespecified analytical strategies. It is therefore important to plan sensitivity analysis to ensure the validity of the assumptions and the robustness of the findings under plausible scenarios. The approaches used for any sensitivity analyses should address the same underlying question or study objective as the initial or primary analysis.

When interim analyses are anticipated, the frequency of analysis, the purpose, and the approach to be used to control Type I error rates are important factors to consider in advance. In terms of design, it is customary to consider the group sequential approach, as it provides operational convenience and efficiency. Stopping trials early for clear efficacy should be considered in the context of improved estimation and additional safety information accrued if the trial continues. However, in certain situations, other adaptive approaches, such as the randomized play-the-winner rule, may also be useful (Rosenberg 1999). In any case, appropriate processes should be put in place for monitoring the study and review of the interim results to ensure the integrity of the trial and credibility of the results (see, e.g., Ellenberg et al. 2002; FDA 2006).

When the treatment effect is positive in a clinical trial the implied inference is about the overall population as defined in the protocol. However, there is growing expectation from regulatory agencies, as well as the medical community and insurers for data on subgroups, defined by relevant patient characteristics, including sex, race, age, and other potential prognostic factors. Subgroup analysis requires caution, especially in confirmatory trials, where the analysis is performed following positive findings in the overall trial population. From a statistical perspective, the main issues concern false positives, the missinterpretation of positive findings in a specific subgroup as confirmatory of a treatment effect within that subgroup, as well as false negatives, due to small sample sizes within subgroups. In situations in which the analyses are preplanned and for confirmatory purposes, suitable statistical methods should be applied to address multiplicity issues. In addition, when there is a confirmatory objective within a subgroup, efforts should be made to design the study with adequate power to detect the subgroup effect. For subgroup analyses intended to generate hypotheses or signal detection for further investigation, alternative approaches have been proposed, including use of modern analytic techniques. A detailed discussion of the approaches may be found, e.g., in Alemayehu et al. (2017) and Dmitrienko et al. (2016).

1.2.5 Reporting and Interpretation of Study Results

To ensure appropriate interpretation and use of trial results, good practices should be followed for the presentation and reporting of the output of statistical analyses. When presenting complex data, graphical displays may be used to highlight important aspects of the findings. Estimated effect sizes should be presented with the associated measures of precision, including standard errors and confidence intervals. For added transparency, any known limitations of the statistical methods used or deviations from planned analyses should be disclosed. In particular, there should be a detailed discussion of measures taken to mitigate common analytical issues such as missing values, outliers, and potential confounding factors. Further, in reporting results from subgroup analyses, there should be a full disclosure of whether the analyses were prespecified, how the subgroups were defined, and the approach used to handle multiplicity (Wang et al. 2007).

1.2.6 Data Quality and Software Validity

The reliability of study results is heavily dependent on the quality of data used for statistical analysis and inference. Therefore, appropriate processes should be instituted to ensure that the study is monitored, and the data processed with high standards throughout the conduct of the trial. When feasible, the data collection and transmission should be accomplished using suitable technology, including electronic data capture tools and modern analytics, to enhance efficiency as well as quality. Further, any software used for various data management tasks, notably data entry, cleaning, and storage, should have appropriate documentation to ascertain the validity and reliability of the trial data (see ICH E3 1996, especially Section 9.6).

1.3 EVOLVING ROLES OF THE STATISTICIAN IN DRUG DEVELOPMENT

It has long been recognized that sound statistical reasoning is critical to ensure the integrity of a clinical trial and the reliability of the accompanying results (Guideline for good Clinical Practice E6 (R1), ICH 1996). Therefore, input from a well-qualified statistician is a requirement in the design, analysis, and reporting of a clinical trial in almost every stage of a clinical development program. As the paradigm for regulatory review and approval evolved, the role of the statistician has also advanced over the years, with increasing visibility and impact across the drug development continuum. In this section, we highlight some of the major activities of the statistician as an integral member of a study team and as a key player in the wider drug development ecosystem.

Historically, the most recognizable responsibility of the statistician, in tandem with data analysis, has been the determination of sample size, since this would have impact on important operational factors such as size of the study, number of participating sites, study duration, and cost. Over time, the statistician's role has expanded and become indispensable in almost every aspect of the trial, ranging from protocol development to participation in investigators meetings and trial result reporting. Much of this expanded role has been driven by the increased importance of the SAP, which is primarily the responsibility of the statistician.

This expanded role has also created further opportunity for the statistician to collaborate with diverse stakeholders, particularly clinicians, data managers, statistical programmers, clinical pharmacologists, regulatory affairs personnel, and regulatory authorities. Accordingly, the statistician is expected to have a good grasp of the end-to-end clinical trial process to provide effective input and to eventually handle potential queries from regulatory bodies relating to relevant aspects of the trial. For example, the statistician's partnership with the clinician requires a thorough understanding of the research hypothesis, the disease area, and the regulatory landscape. In addition, the statistician is expected to have adequate familiarity with the current literature, especially the pertinent guidance documents issued by regulatory bodies (Gerlinger et al. 2012).

In data management, the statistician can help ensure that the data will be captured and cleaned appropriately. In working with statistical programmers, the statistician can provide guidance in the development of programming specifications and codes to generate tables and implement statistical procedures. And, in the course of the reporting of the study results, the statistician can guide the interpretation of the scientific findings with objectivity and fair balance.

The specific roles that the statisticians play may also vary depending on the phase of drug development. For example, a statistician assigned to a Phase I trial may focus on designs appropriate for dose selection, within the constraints of available sample sizes. In late Phase II and Phase III trials, the statistician's responsibilities center not only on the usual tasks relating to trial design, analysis, and reporting, but also on the overall development program and submission strategies. Further, when sponsors interact with regulatory bodies, the statistician is expected to address statistical issues pertaining to almost all aspects of the study.

Besides the usual tasks of design, analysis, and reporting of clinical trials, statisticians also routinely contribute to other areas including process improvement, benefit–risk evaluation, health technology assessment (HTA), cost-effectiveness estimation, business development support, and evaluation and implementation of new technologies. As an integral part of study and submission teams, the statistician is actively engaged in initiatives targeting efficiency, quality, and timeliness of study activities. These tasks may involve development of data standards, streamlining data management operations, or automation of table and listing generation.

With regard to benefit–risk assessment, regulators and pharmaceutical companies around the world frequently use qualitative and quantitative approaches that involve appropriate syntheses of information from clinical trial and other sources in a structured manner. The assessment is often based on multiple factors, including the intended indication, the strength and limitation of the available evidence, and the uncertainties around the benefit and risk estimates (Smith et al. 2017). Therefore, the statistician's role is critical in ensuring the appropriate selection and implementation of standard approaches, and in the interpretation of the results.

Complementing the usual regulatory review process, HTA has a prominent place in many countries for decisions impacting the accessibility of a new drug to patients, especially in influencing its acceptance by payers and other healthcare providers. Indeed, many agencies now require formal submission of data on health economics and outcomes research relating to the value of a treatment option, taking into account such diverse factors as effectiveness, costs, and other measures of utility. The process may require application of both standard and nonstandard statistical techniques and data sources, which are often associated with unique and complex conceptual and practical challenges. For example, in the evaluation of health-related quality of life (HRQOL), an important component of HTA, statisticians may be engaged in the development of the relevant instruments for capturing patient-reported outcomes (PROs), and in addressing conceptual and methodological issues specific to the PROs (Alemayehu and Cappelleri 2012).

Development of biomarkers is another area that requires statistical expertise. Biomarkers can be used as prognostic tools, i.e., to assess disease progression in patients; or for predictive purposes, i.e., identification of subgroups that are more likely to benefit from treatment. Standard statistical techniques are available to analyze routine biomarker data (Fleming and Powers 2012). However, when data cannot readily be analyzed by traditional models, e.g., due to high dimensionality, statisticians can explore the viability of modern machine learning techniques (see, e.g., Swan et al. 2015).

In comparative effectiveness research, meta-analysis and systematic reviews (Brown et al 2011) are often used to generate evidence in support of healthcare decision-making. Traditional meta-analytic approaches consist of pooling data from two or more trials, derived from the literature or other sources, using suitable statistical approaches. When direct evidence is not available from head-to-head RCTs involving all treatment pairs of interest, one often uses network meta-analysis or mixed treatment comparisons. However, the techniques are generally based on certain untestable assumptions, including similarity of experimental conditions and consistency of effects across trials. To strengthen the rigor of the evidence derived from such analyses, statisticians can contribute not only in the synthesis of the information, but also in the development of important guidelines (Liberati et al. 2009).

Regulators are now in the forefront of the efforts to transform the clinical development paradigm, and there are numerous efforts that are spearheaded by various regulatory agencies around the globe. In the US, the *21st Century Cures Act* incorporates several provisions intended to streamline the evidence generation as well as the drug approval processes. The European Medicines Agency (EMA) has as one of its strategic goals the advancement of innovative methods in the development of medicines. Unsurprisingly, the role of the statistician is indispensable in implementing these novel approaches. In adaptive trial designs, for example, whether the goal is to implement adaptive randomization, sample size reestimation, or seamless Phase II/III trial design (Chow and Chang 2008; Stallard and Todd 2010), the effective implementation of the approaches requires application of sound statistical methods and principles. A survey reported in Elsäßer et al. (2014) showed that, while the EMA was generally in favor of adaptive clinical trial designs, there were also instances where the agency provided critical comments, especially concerning multiplicity and bias issues. Therefore, even in some of the simpler cases, it is always advisable for sponsors to engage the appropriate regulatory bodies before implementing these novel approaches.

Recent developments, such as data-sharing initiatives and the digital revolution, provide new opportunities for statisticians to advance evidence generation for critical decision-making. The precompetitive sharing of clinical trial data generated by different pharmaceutical companies can ensure effective use of study information by drug developers and regulatory agencies (Fletcher et al. 2013). In addition, use of modern analytic tools and Big Data can foster the efforts to realize the promise of personalized medicine.

The evolution of the role of statisticians over the years is particularly evident in their involvement in a broad spectrum of strategic tasks. The strategic work ranges from providing critical input in formulating clinical development plans to taking an active part in decision-making in the course of regulatory interactions. In many pharmaceutical companies, statisticians are regular participants in governance bodies and in task forces charged with the development and implementation of processes and best practices to enhance the quality and efficiency of clinical trials.

To effectively execute these enhanced roles, the statistician should develop correspondingly increased strategic, technical, interpersonal, and communication skills. Mehrotra and Gobburu (2016) identify four tenets of effective communications; namely, credibility, decision, style of communication, and knowing the audience. Although their proposal targets pharmacometricians, most of the recommendations also apply to statisticians. To establish credibility, in addition to technical skills, the statistician needs to demonstrate a fairly comprehensive knowledge of the risks and benefits of a whole program, and proven ability to actively engage regulatory bodies and other stakeholders to shape the drug development paradigm. Since the statistician works as a member of an interdisciplinary team, he or she should foster teamwork and cultivate a culture of operating in a matrix or cross-functional environment. This requires following a style of communication that promotes collaboration and understanding the audience.

In general, pharmaceutical statisticians acquire the skills that enable them to be effective in their expanded roles while executing the usual statistical duties that are expected of them. In some instances, targeted training may be provided to strengthen their soft skills. The strategic roles can also be enhanced by developing alternative career paths, with appropriate rewards and incentives (Burger et al. 2012).

1.4 POTENTIAL STATISTICAL ISSUES IN REGULATORY REVIEW

There are several statistical issues that can arise in the course of the review of a submission for a new drug approval. To help establish a common understanding of expectations between regulatory bodies and sponsors, specific guidelines have been developed relating to statistical review and evaluation (FDA 2010). However, despite genuine efforts by sponsors to adhere to good statistical principles and relevant guidance documents, there are almost always questions that arise in the course of the review, requiring additional explanations (Chow and Song 2015). The issues range from data quality to the impact of protocol amendments, interpretation of study results, and independence of data monitoring committees. Next we take a high-level look at some of these issues.

1.4.1 Data Quality

Issues that arise with regard to data quality include missing values, inconsistencies (especially in safety assessment), and validity of instruments used to capture the data. Missing data are particularly important, since the statistical approach used to handle them, and, hence, the reliability of the analysis results, are heavily dependent on the amount of missing data, the variables affected, and whether the missingness is random or not. In addition, the validity of any instrument used to capture data, especially PROs can be of concern. Other data issues may include outliers, or values that are not plausible, and how they were handled. In some instances, fraudulent data may be detected, and may compromise the entire NDA submission (George and Buyse 2015). More generally, the documentation of the data quality control/assurance procedures the sponsor puts in place may also be suggestive of the degree of the reliability of the data included in the submission package (see ICH E3 1996, especially Section 9.6).

1.4.2 Endpoint Definition

In many situations, such as hypertension studies, the choice of outcome measures may not be controversial. However, there are instances when it may be essential to justify the clinical relevance of the outcome measures. According to one study (Sacks et al. 2014), a major reason for non-approval of NDA submissions is unsatisfactory use of endpoints. A few examples mentioned in the paper include, timing of measurement of outcome, interpretation of a successful treatment outcome, and meaningfulness of size of the change. When multiple endpoints are used, lack of consistency in the observed results may also prevent approval. Further, if a composite measure is used to define the primary outcome, the appropriateness of the definition needs to be justified.

1.4.3 Design and Analysis Issues

As outlined in the FDA manual of policies and procedures (FDA 2012), examples of statistical issues that may be cause for concern include integrity of the blinding, randomization, or unplanned interim analyses; sample size and power determination; any modification or change of primary endpoint during conduct of the trial; dropping/adding treatment arms; sample size reestimation; inconsistency of results across subgroups; handling of multiplicity; and justification for non-inferiority designs.

Among the most controversial issues is one relating to inference on multiple hypotheses. According to Westfall and Bretz (2010), this may include adjustment for multiplicity in dose-finding trials, excessive or inadequate control of the type I error probability, or choice of a family of hypotheses concerning primary and secondary study endpoints. The issue of multiplicity may also become equally important when applying a two-stage adaptive design, since it may not often be clear how the overall type I error rate is controlled at a given level of significance.

When sponsors propose non-inferiority designs, with an active control group, but no placebo arm, there are several issues that may arise in the course of regulatory review. One major factor is the justification for the determination of the non-inferiority margin. For example, when the intent is demonstration of effect preservation by the experimental drug, it has been argued that the customary confidence interval approach cannot attain the intended coverage probability exactly, which tends to fluctuate with the sample size (Hung et al. 2003). Further, in the absence of a placebo arm, it is difficult to assess the constancy of the effect of the active control seen in previous trials. In addition, results based on all randomized patients, in which non-compliant subjects are not excluded, could tend to be biased toward non-inferiority (See Section 2.4 for a discussion of non-inferiority designs).

As stated earlier, the use of adaptive methods in clinical development is actively encouraged by regulatory bodies, especially in rare disease research. However, there are critical statistical and operational issues that may be of concern at the review stage. When such designs are implemented for confirmatory trials, in almost all cases, one needs to address the issue of type I error inflation. A related concern may be the reliability of the treatment effect estimate, as well as the potential heterogeneity of the patient population induced by the modifications of trial procedures in the course of the adaptation process (Chow et al. 2005). Indeed, according to a recent study concerning use of adaptive clinical trial designs for European marketing authorization, the most frequent concerns raised by the Committee for Medicinal Products for Human Use/Scientific Advice Working Party (CHMP/SAWP) include inadequate justifications of the proposed adaptation strategy, the control of type I error rate, and the mitigation of the associated bias (Elsäßer et al. 2014). To facilitate the implementation of adaptive designs, Bayesian techniques are often proposed (Berry 2012). However, the use of Bayesian statistics in regulatory submissions is not very common, except in devices and early-phase trials. While the computational issues that limited the wide use of Bayesian methods have largely been resolved, there are still no clear guidelines on the acceptable use of the techniques in confirmatory trials (see Section 2.6 for a discussion of Bayesian statistics).

1.4.4 Evaluation of Safety

Although the focus in the above section has been on efficacy results, there are also important issues that may arise in the approaches used to assess safety data. Customarily, safety results are often presented using simple descriptive statistics and graphical displays. Formal inference may not be appropriate due to lack of adequate power, multiplicity issues, or the *post hoc* nature of safety data analyses. However, descriptive results may lead to misleading interpretation of the findings. For example, when there are unequal follow-up periods for subjects assigned to different treatment groups, the analysis of adverse events may lead to uninterpretable results (Bender et al. 2016). Meta-analysis is often performed to synthesize safety data from multiple studies; however, this also requires addressing issues of heterogeneity and the handling of rare events. The latter is particularly important, since some of the adverse events may not have been observed in some of the studies. It is also important to keep in mind that serious low-incidence adverse effects may not emerge until the drug is marketed to the population at large. Therefore, caution is required in the interpretation of safety data, balancing the potential risk vs. the imperative to bring new medicines to patients that need them.

1.4.5 Analysis Populations and Subgroups

Ideally, the primary analysis should be performed on all randomized subjects. However, that ideal may not be practical for various operational or technical reasons. The study population to be used for the primary analysis may be controversial if any exclusion of patients compromises the benefits of the randomization or the appropriate estimation of the targeted treatment effect. Therefore, any exclusion of randomized patients from the primary analysis should be carefully justified and prespecified in the study protocol. Common reasons for exclusion may include major violation of eligibility criteria, failure to take any trial medication, or the lack of data after randomization. There are also situations that may require specific consideration for the definition of the analysis population to strengthen the interpretability of the results. Examples of scenarios in which patient exclusion may be essential include non-inferiority studies, safety assessment, and fraudulent data from certain sites.

Subgroup analyses are essential to ascertain the risk–benefit of a new drug in special groups defined by demographic or baseline variables. The statistical issues that arise may be both in the definition of the subgroups, as well as in the meaningfulness of the conclusions drawn. The estimate, of course, will vary over subgroups and it may not often be clear if the subgroup-specific estimate is better than the overall estimate for a specific subgroup. Subgroups defined by age, gender, race, or geographic region may be straightforward. However, when other baseline covariates, e.g., biomarkers, are used to define subgroups, the criteria used must be prespecified and the scientific rationale justified. Further, the consistency of the results across subgroup categories should be adequately assessed, and if there is no adequate sample size to do so, this should be indicated. Since such subgroup analyses are exploratory in nature, any intent to make claims based on the results may not be appropriate.

1.4.6 Assessing Interpretation and Reliability of Results

Generally, undue focus on statistical significance, without regard to clinical relevance, and overinterpretation of findings that are not consistent with trial objectives, can be causes for concern during regulatory review. Further, when results are sensitive to departures from model assumptions, or are heavily dependent on analysis populations, the reliability of the primary finding may be called into question. In such situations, the robustness of the findings may need to be justified through extensive sensitivity analyses.

1.5 CONCLUDING REMARKS

In this chapter we provided a high-level account of the interplay between statistics and regulatory science. While drug development involves the collaborative efforts of different disciplines, it is noted that statistics and statisticians play a unique role throughout the continuum of the development and approval processes. In particular, the judicious assessment of a new drug with respect to its safety and efficacy requires the effective implementation of basic principles of good statistical practice, encapsulated in regulatory guidelines and other related documents.

In consonance with the changing regulatory and healthcare landscapes, the role of the statistician has evolved over the years, with increasing impact and visibility. In addition to their traditional tasks of designing, analyzing, and reporting of clinical trials, statisticians are now active partners in major decision-making, ranging from formulation of development plans to indispensable engagement in initiatives intended to enhance efficiency and productivity.

The diminishing number of drugs approved, coupled with the skyrocketing healthcare cost, has already made it imperative to explore new paradigms for evidence generation and regulatory approval. Thus, Big Data, modern analytics, and precision medicine will undoubtedly continue to present interesting challenges and opportunities both to regulators and statisticians. In subsequent chapters, some of the topics and issues alluded to in this chapter will be addressed in greater detail, with emphasis on those areas that are deemed critical to statistics–regulatory interaction and to enhancing the impact of statistics in the drug approval process.

BIBLIOGRAPHY

Alemayehu, D., Cappelleri, J. C. (2012) Conceptual and analytical considerations toward the use of patient-reported outcomes in personalized medicine. *American Health and Drug Benefits*. 5: 310–317.

Alemayehu, D., Chen, Y., Markatou, M. (2017) A comparative study of subgroup identification methods for differential treatment effect: Performance metrics and recommendations. *Statistical Methods in Medical Research*. 27(12): 3658–3678. 096228021771057. 10.1177/0962280217710570.

Bender, R., Beckmann, L., Lange, S. (2016) Biometrical issues in the analysis of adverse events within the benefit assessment of drugs. *Pharmaceutical Statistics*. 15(4): 292–296.

Berry, D. A. (2012) Adaptive clinical trials in oncology. *Nature Reviews Clinical Oncology*. 9: 199–207.

Berry, D. A. (2015) The brave new world of clinical cancer research: Adaptive biomarker-driven trials integrating clinical practice with clinical research. *Molecular Oncology*. 9: 951–959.

Boutron, I., Guillet, L., Estellat, C., Moher, D., Hrobjartsson, A., Ravaud, P. (2006) Reporting methods of blinding in randomized trials assessing pharmacological treatments: A systematic review. *PLoS Medicine*. 3(10): 1931–1939.

Brown, S. R., Gregory, W. M., Twelves, C. J., Buyse, M., Collinson, F., Parmar, M., Seymour, M. T., Brown, J. M. (2011) Designing phase II trials in cancer: A systematic review and guidance. *British Journal of Cancer*. 105: 194–199. pmid: 21712822.

Burger, H. U., Driessen, S., Fletcher, C., Gerlinger, C., Branson, M. (2012) Roles and career paths for statisticians in today's pharmaceutical industry. EFSPI Report.

Chow, S.-C., Chang, M. (2008) Adaptive design methods in clinical trials – A review. *Orphanet Journal of Rare Diseases*. 3: 11.

Chow, S.-C., Chang, M., Pong, A. (2005) Statistical consideration of adaptive methods in clinical development. *Journal of Biopharmaceutical Statistics*.15(4): 575–591. DOI: 10.1081/BIP-200062277

Chow, S.-C., Song, F. (2015) On controversial statistical issues in clinical research. Open Access. *Journal of Clinical Trials*. 7: 43–51.

Dmitrienko, A., Muysers, M., Fritsch, A., Lipkovich, I. (2016) General guidance on exploratory and confirmatory subgroup analysis in late-stage clinical trials. *Journal of Biopharmaceutical Statistics*. 26(1): 71–98. DOI: 10.1080/10543406.2015.1092033.

Donner, A., Klar, N. (2004) Pitfalls of and controversies in cluster randomization trials. *American Journal of Public Health*. 94(3): 416–422.

Ellenberg, S., Fleming, T., DeMets, D. (2002) *Data Monitoring Committees in Clinical Trials: A Practical Perspective*. Chichester: John Wiley & Sons.

Elsäßer, A., Regnstrom, J., Vetter, T., Koenig, F., Hemmings, R. J., Greco, M., Papaluca-Amati, M., Posch, M. (2014) Adaptive clinical trial designs for European marketing authorization: A survey of scientific advice letters from the European Medicines Agency. *Trials*. 15: 383. DOI: 10.1186/1745-6215-15-383.

European Agency for the Evaluation of Medicinal Products (EMEA) ICH Topic E6 (1996) Good clinical practice. London: European Agency for the Evaluation of Medicinal Products; July 1996.

European Agency for the Evaluation of Medicinal Products (EMEA) ICH Topic E9 (1998) Statistical principles for clinical trials. London: European Agency for the Evaluation of Medicinal Products; February 1998.

EMA (2002, 2006) Point to Consider on Methodological Issues in Confirmatory Clinical Trials with Flexible Design and Analysis Plan. The European Agency for the Evaluation of Medicinal Products Evaluation of Medicines for Human Use. CPMP/EWP/2459/02, London, UK.

Finfer, S., Bellomo, R. (2009) Why publish statistical analysis plans? *Critical Care and Resuscitation*. 11(1): 5–6.

Fleming, T. R., Powers, J. H. (2012) Biomarkers and surrogate endpoints in clinical trials. *Statistics in Medicine.* 31: 2973–2974.

Fletcher, C., Driessen, S., Burger, H. U., Gerlinger, C., Biesheuvel, E. (2013) European Federation of Statisticians in the Pharmaceutical Industry's position on access to clinical trial data. *Pharmaceutical Statistics.* 12 (6): 333–336.

Gamble, C., Krishan, A., Stocken, D., Lewis, S., Juszczak, E., Doré, C., Williamson, P. R., Altman, D. G., Montgomery, A., Lim, P., Berlin, J., Senn, S., Day, S., Barbachano, Y., Loder, E. (2017) Guidelines for the content of statistical analysis plans in clinical trials. *Journal of American Medical Association.* 318(23): 2337–2343. DOI: 10.1001/jama.2017.18556.

George, S. L., Buyse, M. (2015) Data fraud in clinical trials. *Clinical Investigation.* 5(2): 161–173. http://doi.org/10.4155/cli.14.116.

Gerlinger, C., Edler, L., Friede, T., Kieser, M., Nakas, C. T., Schumacher, M., Seldrup, J., Victor, N. (2012) Considerations on what constitutes a "Qualified Statistician" in regulatory guidelines. *Statistics in Medicine.* 31: 1303–1305.

Hung, H. M. J., Wang, S.-J., Tsong, Y., Lawrence, J., O'Neil, R. T. (2003) Some fundamental issues with non-inferiority testing in active controlled trials. *Statistics in Medicine.* 22(2), January 30: 213–225. DOI: 10.1002/sim.1315.

International Conference on Harmonization of Technical Requirements for Registration of Pharmaceuticals for Human Use (1998) *ICH Harmonized Tripartite Guideline: Statistical Principles for Clinical Trials E9.* London: European Medicines Agency.

International Conference of Harmonization (1996) ICH guideline for good clinical practice E6 (R1). www.ich.org/products/guidelines/efficacy/article/efficacy-guidelines.html (accessed December 16, 2014).

International Conference of Harmonization (1996) ICH guideline for industry structure and content of clinical study reports (E3). www.fda.gov/regulatory-information/search-fda-guidance-documents/e3-structure-and-content-clinical-study-reports (accessed July 19, 2020).

Kramar, A., Potvin, D., Hill C. (1996) Multistage designs for phase II clinical trials: Statistical issues in cancer research. *British Journal of Cancer.* 74(8): 1317–1320.

Lara, P. N., Redman, M. W. (2012) The hazards of randomized phase II trials. *Annals of Oncology.* 23(1): 7–9.

Liberati, A., Altman, D. G., Tetzlaff, J., Mulrow, C., Gøtzsche, P. C., Ioannidis, J. P. A., Clarke, M., Devereaux, P. J., Kleijnen, J., Mohe, D., the PRISMA Group (2009) The PRISMA Statement for reporting systematic reviews and meta-analyses of studies that evaluate health care interventions: Explanation and elaboration. *Annals of Internal Medicine.* 151: W-65–W-94.

Maclure, M. (2009) Explaining pragmatic trials to pragmatic policy-makers. *Canadian Medical Association Journal.* 180: 1001–1003.

Mehrotra, S., Gobburu, J. (2016) Communicating to influence drug development and regulatory decisions: A tutorial. *CPT: Pharmacometrics & Systems Pharmacology.* 5(4): 163–172. DOI: 10.1002/psp4.12073.

Mentz, R. J., Hernandez, A. F., Berdan, L. G., Rorick, T., O'Brien, E. C., Ibarra, J. C., Curtis, L. H., Peterson, E. D. (2016) Good clinical practice guidance and pragmatic clinical trials: Balancing the best of both worlds. *Circulation.* 133: 872–880.

Patsopoulos, N. A. (2011) A pragmatic view on pragmatic trials. *Dialogues in Clinical Neuroscience.* 13: 217–224.

Postel-Vinay, S., Aspeslagh, S., Lanoy, E., Robert, C., Soria, J.-C., Marabelle, A. (2016) Challenges of Phase 1 clinical trials evaluating immune checkpoint targeted antibodies. *Annals of Oncology.* 27(2): 214–224. doi:10.1093/annonc/mdv550: official journal of the European Society for Medical Oncology / ESMO. 27. 10.1093/annonc/mdv550.

Renfro, L. A., Sargent, D. J. (2017) Statistical controversies in clinical research: Basket trials, umbrella trials, and other master protocols: A review and examples. *Annals of Oncology.* 28(1): 34–43.

Roehr, B. (2013) The appeal of large simple trials. *British Medical Journal.* 346: f1317.

Rosenberg, W. F. (1999) Randomized play-the-winner clinical trials: Review and recommendations. *Controlled Clinical Trials.* 20: 328–342.

Sacks, L. V., Shamsuddin, H. H., Yasinskaya, Y. I., Bouri, K., Lanthier, M. L., Sherman, R. E. (2014) Scientific and regulatory reasons for delay and denial of FDA approval of initial applications for new drugs, 2000-2012. *Journal of American Medical Association.* 311(4): 378–384. DOI: 10.1001/jama.2013.282542.

Schultz, K. F., Grimes, D. A. (2002) Generation of allocation sequences in randomized trials: Chance, not choice. *Lancet.* 359: 515–519.

Sibbald, B., Roland, M. (1998) Understanding controlled trials. Why are randomised controlled trials important? *British Medical Journal.* 316: 201.

Smith, M., Benattia, I., Strauss, C., Bloss, L., Jiang, Q. (2017) Structured benefit-risk assessment across the product lifecycle: Practical considerations. *Therapeutic Innovation & Regulatory Science.* 51. DOI: 10.1177/2168479017696272.

Stallard, N., Todd, S. (2010) Seamless phase II/III design. *Statistical Methods in Medical Research.* 20(6): 623–634.

Swan, A. L., Stekel, D. J., Hodgman, C., Allaway, D., Alqahtani, M. H., Mobasheri, A., Bacardit, J. (2015) A machine learning heuristic to identify biologically relevant and minimal biomarker panels from omics data. *BMC Genomics.* 16(Suppl 1): S2. http://doi.org/10.1186/1471-2164-16-S1-S2.

Wang, R., Lagakos, S. W., Ware, J. H., Hunter, D. J., Drazen, J. M. (2007) Statistics in medicine – Reporting of subgroup analyses in clinical trials. *New England Journal of Medicine*. 357: 2189–2194.

US FDA (2010) Guidance for industry: Adaptive design clinical trials for drugs and biologics. Washington DC.

US FDA (2012) Statistical review and evaluation. Clinical studies. www.fda.gov/downloads/aboutfda/centersoffices/officeofmedicalproductsandtobacco/cder/manualofpoliciesprocedures/ucm313814.pdf.

US FDA Center for Drug Evaluation and Research (2010) MAPP 6010.3 Rev. 1: Good review practice: Clinical review template.

US FDA Guidance for Clinical Trial Sponsors (2006) Establishment and operation of clinical trial data monitoring committees. Silver Spring: US FDA.

Westfall, P., Bretz, F. (2010) Multiplicity in clinical trials. In: Chow S.-C., editor. *Encyclopedia of Biopharmaceutical Statistics*. 3rd ed. New York: Taylor and Francis: 889–896.

World Health Organization (2002) WHO handbook for good clinical research practice (GCP) guidance for implementation. http://apps.who.int/prequal/info_general/documents/GCP/gcp1.pdf (accessed December 15, 2014).

CHAPTER 2

Selected Statistical Topics of Regulatory Importance

2.1 INTRODUCTION

This chapter provides a detailed discussion of major statistical issues that commonly arise in the course of drug development and regulatory interactions. The section on multiplicity outlines measures that should be taken to ensure the validity of inferential results that are intended to be the basis for regulatory decision-making. In a separate section, a thorough review of best practices is provided to handle missing values, which are ubiquitous in clinical trials, with special reference to pertinent guidelines and the emergent topic of estimands. While superiority trials are common to support drug approval, there are situations where it is necessary to conduct non-inferiority studies. The regulatory requirements and underlying principles of such trials are summarized, and suggestions are provided relating to the salient points to be considered for both efficacy and safety assessment. In light of the increasing focus to accelerate drug development by improved efficiency, a summary of a few of the commonly used novel approaches is provided, including adaptive and flexible designs, enrichment studies, and studies conducted under the so-called master protocols. Other topics of regulatory and statistical import covered in this chapter include Bayesian approaches, issues with subgroup analysis, biomarkers, and the assessment of benefits and risks of pharmaceutical products.

2.2 MULTIPLICITY

The issue of multiplicity refers in general to the inflation of the Type 1 error in the interpretation of clinical trial results. Controlling the probability of falsely concluding a treatment effect is of special concern to regulators and hence multiplicity is often an important statistical issue in the review of confirmatory clinical trials. The question of multiplicity can arise in many ways. We will address three main areas of multiplicity in the regulatory setting: multiple primary endpoints and secondary endpoints with the potential to be included in the product label; multiple testing in the course of the study with the purpose to stop for positive results (interim analyses); and subgroup analyses. Within the multiple endpoint section, we will briefly discuss other aspects of a study design that can inflate the Type 1 error rate. Further detailed discussions of multiplicity may be found, e.g., in Alosh et al. (2014), Dmitrienko et al. (2013), and Huque et al. (2013), among others.

2.2.1 Multiple Endpoints

Statistical hypothesis testing in a regulatory setting involves the calculation under the null hypothesis of the probability that the observed treatment effect on a specific variable is due to chance alone. In a randomized study, if this probability (p-value) is low, the null hypothesis (usually that the treatment effect is 0) is rejected and a treatment effect is established. If only one primary variable is used to establish a treatment effect, then the requirement that $p < \alpha$ controls the probability of incorrectly concluding a treatment effect at α. The issue of multiplicity of endpoints refers to the clinical trial setting where more than one variable is used to establish a treatment effect. The chances of obtaining at least one p-value below α increase with the number of endpoints. For example, the probability under the null hypothesis that at least one p-value is less than 0.05 for three independent hypotheses is $1 - (0.95)^3 = 0.14$. Thus, regulators cannot accept a level α test for each variable if the goal is to rule out incorrectly concluding a treatment effect (Type I error) at an overall probability of α.

In a good clinical trial design, there should be a set of primary endpoints and level of significance specified in the protocol that will determine whether the study has met its objective or not. The set of primary endpoints consists of the measures that establish the effectiveness of the drug in order to support regulatory action. When there is more than one primary endpoint and an effect on any of the endpoints is sufficient to establish the drug's effectiveness, then the rate of falsely concluding the drug is effective is increased over the Type I error used for each hypothesis. Consequently, if the goal is to control the probability that a chance finding is misinterpreted as treatments effect at level α, then an adjustment must be made to the significance tests of the individual variables.

There are many statistical methods to control for overall Type I error in the setting of multiple primary endpoints. Commonly used procedures are Bonferroni, Hochberg, Holms, and general sequential testing procedures. In the Bonferroni procedure, α is typically divided evenly among the total number of variables T and the individual p-values are compared to α/T. Holms and Hochberg are both multistep procedures where the observed p-values are compared to α/T, $\alpha/(T-1)$, …, α. The Holms procedure begins with the smallest observed p-value compared to α/T and continues to larger p-values until the observed p-value is not significant. The Hochberg procedure begins with the largest p-value compared to α and continues to lower p-values until significance is reached in which case all variables with lower p-values are also significant. General sequential testing procedures allow for a prespecified ordering of the variables and carrying forward any unused α.

Multiple-testing procedures have been well-described in the literature (e.g., Dmitrienko et al. 2013; Proschan and Waclawiw 2000) and it is not the purpose to review them here, or to recommend one procedure over the other. The multiple comparison procedure should be prespecified and selected in the context of the specific protocol objectives and the expected treatment effects on the multiple primary endpoints. In some cases there may be a regulatory requirement to show that the treatment is effective on more than one endpoint. For example, a treatment for Alzheimer's disease might have to show effectiveness on both a measure of cognitive function and on a measure of quality of life. In this case no multiple comparison procedure is required.

In clinical trials it would be remiss not to assess many measures of change in the patient's disease state outside of the primary endpoint(s). While these measures are not sufficient in and of themselves to establish effectiveness in the disease under study, it may be important to include them in the package insert given that the primary endpoint(s) have established a sufficient basis for approval. The analysis and interpretation of a drug's effectiveness on these secondary endpoints may also require a multiple comparison procedure to control overall Type I error at a prespecified level. Positive results (nominal statistical significance) from a list of secondary endpoints without Type 1 error control would not be enough evidence to conclude a treatment effect and not likely to lead to inclusion in the package insert or in promotional material. There are small differences in the FDA guidance and the EMA guidance on Type 1 control of secondary endpoints. FDA guidance (FDA 2017b) states: "This includes controlling the Type I error rate within and between the primary and secondary endpoint families"; whereas the EMA guidance (EMA 2017b) states:

> *Including secondary endpoints in a multiple testing procedure (e.g., a "hierarchy") is therefore not mandated, but permits a quantification of the risk of a type I error regarding these endpoints, which may lend support that an individual result is sufficiently reliable when included in the Summary of Product Characteristics.*

Thus, Type 1 error control by a multiple comparison procedure on secondary endpoints is extremely useful from the sponsor's perspective in order to potentially get the information in the package insert and is extremely useful from the regulator's perspective to control the misinterpretation of a chance finding as a treatment effect. It is recommended that important secondary endpoints for potential label implications should be specified in the protocol along with an appropriate multiple comparison procedure to control Type I error at α.

Some additional important points to consider from a statistical–regulatory perspective regarding Type 1 error control are:

- The set of primary and secondary endpoints are often referred to as families of endpoints. While regulatory agencies require Type 1 error control for both the primary and secondary families (family-wise error rate, FWER), a stronger study-wide error rate may be required. This is accomplished by controlling both the primary- and secondary-family error rate at α and testing the secondary family of endpoints only if the treatment effect is established within the primary endpoints. This is a specific example of the general class of "gatekeeping strategies" for controlling study-wide error rate.
- When there is more than one primary endpoint the effect of the specific multiplicity procedure on power should be considered and included in the determination of the study sample size.

- An important type of multiplicity involves the analysis of the individual components of composite or multicriteria endpoints. When there are competing outcomes of interest for use as a primary endpoint, it may be advisable to combine them into a single variable or score. In addition to avoiding multiplicity issues, the so-called composite endpoints may be defined to gain power when the incidence rate on the components is anticipated to be low. In some cases, e.g., patient-reported outcomes (PROs), a multicomponent endpoint may be collapsed into a single overall score using suitable summary statistics, such as the sum or average across the individual domain scores. Recently, alternative approaches have been proposed for defining and analyzing composite endpoints. Examples include the win ratio, proposed by Pocock et al. (2012), and the joint rank test of Finkelstein and Schoenfeld (1999). In general, when the composite endpoint is significant, it may be worthwhile to assess the effect of treatment on the components separately. Here a multiplicity procedure should be specified to control falsely concluding a treatment effect on any given component of the composite endpoint. There is also the regulatory interest that the observed benefit of the study drug is not unduly influenced by one or more endpoints of lower relevance in the composite endpoint.
- In the above discussion, the focus has been on hypothesis testing. Although confidence intervals are generally used to specify the magnitude of the treatment effect and the associated degree of precision, in some cases they may be used to test hypotheses. When that is the case, it would be appropriate to ensure that multiplicity issues are addressed accordingly.
- Multiple endpoints are not the only source of multiplicity in clinical trials that can lead to an inflated Type 1 error rate. For example, a confirmatory clinical trial may have more than one dose group where at least one dose must be significantly better than placebo. An oncology study could consist of more than one type of cancer or even the same cancer with different predetermined cell markers, and the objective is for approval of either type of cancer or cell type. These multiple objectives can inflate Type 1 error. When multiple primary endpoints are included in these more complex designs, the control of Type 1 error can be more difficult. However, from the regulators' perspective any confirmatory conclusion regarding an indication (or claim within the package insert) must have Type 1 error control to protect against a false positive statement.

The above discussion on multiplicity in the context of regulatory decision-making is from a hypothesis testing, frequentist approach to statistics, which is the viewpoint embedded in ICH E9 Statistical Principles for Clinical Trials (1998) and both the FDA and EMA guidance on multiplicity issues. While ICH E9 is dominated by the frequentist approach, it does not rule out Bayesian approaches. With the increasing use of more complex, multi-objective clinical trials, as well as adaptive and even more innovative clinical trial designs, the use of Bayesian methods to inform regulatory decision-making may increase in the future. However, for now the dominant regulatory perspective is for the sponsor to control the probability of a study falsely "winning" (concluding a treatment effect) given all the ways of winning as defined within the protocol.

2.2.2 Multiple Testing Over the Course of the Study

Interim analyses of an ongoing clinical trial can be conducted for many reasons, particularly with the emerging methods of adaptive designs. We discuss interim analysis from the more traditional perspective of sequential designs where interim analyses are conducted for the purpose of stopping the study for a positive efficacy result. Interim analyses are another source of multiplicity that inflates Type I error α in clinical trials if not taken into account. Clearly, the more often the primary null hypothesis is tested with accruing data, the higher is the probability that a true null will be rejected leading to a false conclusion of a treatment effect. Consequently, regulators require that the sum of the probabilities of rejecting a true null at each interim analysis is $\leq \alpha$. For example, suppose the study is designed to have two interim analyses and a final analysis with the potential to stop the study at either of the two interim analyses for positive results. Let

p_1 = the probability of rejecting a true null hypothesis at the first interim analysis

p_2 = the probability of rejecting a true null hypothesis at the second interim analysis and that it was not rejected at the first interim analysis

p_F = the probability of rejecting a true null hypothesis at the final analysis and that it was not rejected at the first and second interim analyses

Then a regulatory requirement for this interim analysis procedure is that $p_1 + p_2 + p_F \leq \alpha$. The actual values for the probabilities should be determined by the sponsor in consultation with the regulatory agencies based on study consideration. The methods for controlling Type 1 error in designs with interim analyses fall under the general terminology of α-spending functions.

Prior to the introduction of α-spending functions there were specific group-sequential-testing procedures established for equal space testing. The equal spacing refers to the information time τ_i, i.e., the proportion of the total information at the end of the study available at the time of the ith interim analysis. The two prominent ones were the Pocock procedure (Pocock 1977) and the O'Brien–Fleming procedure (O'Brien and Fleming 1979). The Pocock procedure is characterized by a constant critical rejection value at each interim analysis while the O'Brien–Fleming procedure is characterized by critical rejection values that are inversely proportional to the square-root of the information time. Table 2.1 illustrates the Pocock and O'Brien–Fleming critical values for 3 equally spaced interim analyses and one-side $\alpha = 0.025$.

While both procedures preserve overall Type 1 error at α, they do so in different ways. The O'Brien–Fleming procedure is stricter at earlier interim analyses where the information fraction is relatively small, but preserves much of the α for the final analysis where the rejection value is close to the fixed-sample-size rejection value of 1.96. In contrast the Pocock procedure, with constant rejection values, allows for a better chance to reject the null hypothesis at earlier interim analyses but preserves a smaller amount of α for the final analysis.

In addition to the control of Type 1 error, two necessary features of the O'Brien–Fleming, Pocock, and similar procedures are the requirements that the maximum number of scheduled analyses must be determined prior to the onset of the trial and that the interim analyses are equally spaced, with respect to information fraction τ. As a way to relax these restrictions as well as to provide a uniform way to view interim analyses and the allocation of

TABLE 2.1 Rejection Values (RV) and Nominal p-values for O'Brien–Fleming and Pocock Procedures with 3 Interim Analyses, One-side $\alpha = 0.025$.

	O'Brien–Fleming		Pocock	
τ	RV	p	RV	P
1/3	3.438	0.0003	2.289	0.0110
2/3	2.431	0.0075	2.289	0.0110
1	1.985	0.0235	2.289	0.0110

α, Lan and DeMets (1983) developed the method of the alpha-spending function. An α-spending function, $\alpha(\tau)$, relates the cumulative spending of α as a function of the information fraction τ. At the beginning of the study $\alpha(\tau) = 0$ and at the end of trial $\alpha(\tau) = \alpha$. Neither the times nor the number of analyses need to be specified in advance. Only the functional form of $\alpha(\tau)$ must be specified. Thus, the Lan–DeMets α-spending function method generalizes the group-sequential method that spends α at discrete predetermined times. The use of a prespecified continuous α-spending function allows for the number and timing of the interim analyses to remain unspecified.

The spending of α can be thought of as falling into two broad categories; conservative, which preserves much of α for the end of the trial, and aggressive, which spends greater amounts of α earlier in the trial. These approaches are exemplified by the O'Brien–Fleming procedure and the Pocock procedure. Consequently, spending functions are often referred to as an O'Brien–Fleming-type or Pocock-type spending function.

Interim analyses and the α-spending function have to be considered in the regulatory context. In confirmatory clinical trials the number of interim analyses is often limited to a single interim analysis for the purpose of stopping the trial for futility or strong efficacy results. However, it is often not advisable to stop a trial early for efficacy because additional safety data may be desirable from the regulatory perspective or more information regarding subgroups or secondary measures of the disease is desirable. From a practical perspective, the statistical planning for an interim analysis often reduces to selecting p_1, the probability of rejecting a true null hypothesis at the interim analysis and then determining p_F, the probability of rejecting a true null hypothesis at the final analysis and that it was not rejected at the interim analyses. If $p_1 + p_F \leq \alpha$, then this is a discrete spending function that controls Type 1 error at α. Numerical integration or simulation for discrete probability distributions where a normal approximation may not be good can be used to obtain the probability p_F. The actual timing of the interim analysis can be decided after the trial begins. It is strongly recommended that the sponsor obtain agreement with regulators on any interim analysis.

2.3 MISSING VALUES AND ESTIMANDS

2.3.1 General Considerations

Missing data invariably occur in clinical trials and are a main area of regulatory scrutiny in the review process. The issue of missing data has recently been subsumed within the concept of an estimand, which will be addressed in Section 2.3.5. While there are several conditions in which missingness may occur, the one that we are most concerned with is the case involving patients who discontinue the study and are lost-to-follow-up. If not handled properly, results based on incomplete data are likely to be misleading, often associated with bias in favor of a new treatment under study (ICH E9, 1998). Excluding missing values may result in the underestimation of variability of estimators and reduction of the statistical power of tests, thereby compromising the validity of the accompanying inferential results. Further, arbitrarily excluding study subjects adversely impacts the benefits of randomization, intended to ensure comparability of treatment groups as well as the representativeness of the population defined by the protocol inclusion and exclusion criteria. In short, missingness is likely to be informative and consequently, efforts should be made to minimize the occurrence of missing data at the design and conduct stages of a trial, and to implement appropriate analytical strategies to buttress the reliability of the results. Recently, several documents have been issued by regulatory authorities to establish minimum requirements to assure the validity of trial conclusions drawn from data with incomplete information (see, e.g., the guidelines from European Medicines Agency and the US FDA-mandated panel report from National Research Council (NRC) (FDA 2010)).

There are several reasons why data may be incomplete, some of which may be attributable to the treatment under study. Examples of the latter include missing data as a result of inability or unwillingness of patients to continue in a study because the treatment is not beneficial, lacks efficacy, or causes undesirable side effects. In other cases, the reason for incompleteness of data may be completely unrelated to the treatment under study. For example, patients may drop out of a study as a result of changes in their physical address, family status, or other personal situation not related to their health. In either case, the incompleteness of the data may have considerable impact on the credibility and reliability of the accompanying study results.

When dealing with missing values, the interrelated factors that get increased attention in the course of regulatory assessment include the reason for missingness, the proportion of missingness, the demographics of subjects who dropout from the study, and the approach used for the analysis and reporting of the data. The rigor in which missingness issues are addressed and the measures taken to minimize any bias favoring the experimental agent are critical factors in the assessment of the strength of the evidence submitted in support of the benefit of the new intervention.

Depending on the assumptions made about the mechanism generating the missing values, there are alternative approaches for analyzing the data. In the choice of a suitable approach, it is generally advisable to look for methods that minimize potential bias in favor of the experimental drug and that do not tend to underestimate the variability of the treatment effect estimates. In most instances, the assumption the analyst makes about the missingness may not be objectively testable. So, irrespective of the method chosen, it is essential to validate the reliability of the results through appropriately planned sensitivity analyses.

Missing values cannot be fully avoided in clinical trials. Further, there is no analytical strategy that can conclusively eliminate the potential bias associated with the missing values. Therefore, one pragmatic approach is to minimize the occurrence of missing values by implementing preventive measures, both during the design stage and in the course of the conduct of the trial (Little et al. 2012). In planning mitigating measures, some of the factors to consider include the length of the trial, complexity of the protocol in terms of the schedule of study procedures, and patient adherence, as well as the use of technology to capture study endpoints. Other relevant considerations include effective communication with investigator sites and study participants regarding the importance of remaining in the study, frequent data monitoring, and real-time data-quality assessment (O'Neill and Temple 2012).

In the rest of this section we will review the types of mechanisms that generate missing data, and summarize commonly used analytical approaches, with emphasis on models for longitudinal and other standard techniques. We will give a brief overview of the current thinking on estimands and the relationship to the problem of missingness, and outline pertinent aspects of the concept that require further elucidation.

2.3.2 Missingness Mechanisms

As pointed out earlier, the mechanism that generates missing values may be related to the study drug or it may be a random phenomenon. In the literature, three types of missingness mechanisms are frequently referenced, depending on whether the mechanism is associated with the observed or unobserved outcomes and other background variables (see, e.g., Diggle and Kenward 1994). Some of the ideas discussed below are especially germane to the special case when the design of a study involves taking repeated measurements on subjects over time.

When the missingness is independent of the subject's responses and other attributes, it is referred to as missing completely at random (MCAR). In this case one may assume that the subjects with missing data are a random sample of all the subjects. A case in point is when a study participant is lost to follow up due to the subject's change in location for reasons unrelated to the disease or treatment. On the other hand, if the missingness depends only on observed data, then it may be classified as missing at random (MAR). This arises, for example, when collected data suggest that the reason a patient dropped out of a study is because either the drug did not improve the patient's condition, or the drug turned out to be toxic. When this mechanism applies, it may be safe to assume that the unobserved or missing data follow the same distribution as those observed values in subjects who have complete information and share the same observed measurements. The MAR assumption implies that after conditioning on observed variables the missingness can be assumed to be MCAR. When the underlying assumptions can be justified, MCAR and MAR scenarios, sometimes referred to as "ignorable," permit application of certain statistical models that yield valid results.

A more difficult, but plausible situation, is one in which the missingness depends on the unobserved response measurements or cannot completely be characterized by the observed information. Often referred to as non-ignorable, or missing not at random (MNAR), this case requires caution, and is generally addressed by sensitivity analyses after an MAR analysis.

There is no formal approach to establish the mechanism by which missing values are generated. In particular, MCAR and MAR are generally untestable, and MNAR is purely speculative. However, as a best practice, one should perform exploratory data analysis to understand the pattern and nature of the missing values. Some simple techniques may include summarizing the frequency and reasons for missing values by study drug and over time; and evaluating and comparing outcome measures as well as other important factors such as demographics, for patients with complete data against those with incomplete observations. To identify any potential association between observed variables and the missing mechanism, one may also perform a suitable model, such as penalized logistic regression, with the missing indicator as the dependent variable. Potential predictors may include safety variables, baseline characteristics, and earlier responses.

2.3.3 Approaches for Missing Data

There are alternative approaches for handling missing data during the analysis phase. The choice of a primary method should, however, be made *a priori*, considering the design of the study, outcome measures, and current regulatory requirements. In general, methods based on MCAR or MNAR assumptions may not be defensible for use in primary analysis. However, the latter may be used in sensitivity analysis concerning the robustness of MAR-based methods, which are commonly implemented for primary analyses.

For the reasons discussed earlier, complete case analysis cannot be justified for the primary analysis, especially in confirmatory trials. It may, however, be considered in early phases of drug development for exploratory purposes or as supportive analysis to confirm the sensitivity of conclusions drawn based on other approaches.

A simple method of handling missing data is the so-called hot-deck imputation, which involves replacing a missing value with a suitable observed value obtained from a matched group of study subjects. Matching may be accomplished using predefined variables and score functions, such as propensity scores (Rosenbaum and Rubin 1983) and the Mahalanobis distance. Since this approach assumes MAR, conditional on the matching variables, the impact of any unobserved variables on the robustness of the results cannot be fully assessed. A high-level overview of the approach may be found, for example, in Andridge and Little (2010).

With longitudinal data involving dropouts, an imputation approach is to carry forward a previously observed value. This approach was commonly used and accepted by regulatory authorities in the past but less so currently due to likely biases in the estimation. Other variations include the best observation or baseline observation (BOCF) or the worst observation (WOCF) carried-forward schemes. When the primary objective of the study is to estimate a treatment effect at the end of a fixed treatment duration, the last observation carried-forward (LOCF) approach is dependent on the assumption of constant disease status after the last observed data; therefore, it can only be applied in the unrealistic case of MCAR and it may lead to bias in cases of MAR or MNAR scenarios. However, if one is interested in estimating a "real-world" treatment effect and the dropout pattern is assumed to represent the real-world performance of the treatment then the last observation yields a valid estimate of real-world performance. Thus, the clinical question being addressed relates to the emerging concept of a valid "estimand" (Section 2.3.5). BOCF, which uses the baseline observation as the final response, is often based on the assumption that a patient withdrew from the trial because of lack of benefit or due to treatment-emergent adverse events. When there are other reasons why patients might withdraw from the trial, the approach would not be reliable (Liu-Seifert et al. 2010).

In general, single imputation methods are likely to lead to incorrect standard errors and, hence, incorrect inferential results, since the error associated with the imputed values is not fully accounted for when performing complete case analysis with the imputed values. Therefore, it is customary to use alternative approaches, such as multiple imputation and likelihood-based inference.

Multiple imputation, first introduced by Rubin (1987), involves imputing each missing value many times, with a view to generating a between-imputation variance component. These data sets, consisting of the multiple-imputed values, are subsequently analyzed using appropriate procedures for complete data. The results from the different data sets are then combined. The approach results in valid hypothesis tests and confidence intervals, which are performed incorporating the uncertainty due to the imputed values.

Several methods are available for computing the imputed values in the above framework, depending on the variable types and missing-data pattern. In general, these imputation methods depend on a MAR assumption. In the case of continuous data, with monotone missing pattern, for example, Rubin (1987) proposes the use of a parametric regression method under multivariate normality or a nonparametric approach based on propensity scores (see, e.g., Lavori, Dawson, and Shera 1995). For a categorical variable with monotone missing patterns, one may implement a logistic-regression model or the discriminant function method. With arbitrary missing-data pattern, imputation may be performed using Markov chain Monte Carlo (MCMC), assuming multivariate normality (Schafer 1997). Other approaches include a fully conditional specification (FCS) method (van Buuren 2007), which assumes a joint distribution for all variables.

Alternatively, likelihood-based methods can be applied under MCAR or MAR assumptions, conditional on observed outcome measurements and baseline covariates. The approaches do not involve explicit creation of imputed values but involve implicit imputations for missing values. One such an approach is the *expectation-maximization* (EM) algorithm (Mallinckrodt 2003), which is an iterative process involving expectation and maximization steps. Informally, the algorithm consists of first estimating the parameters of the model on the basis of complete data, which in turn is used to estimate the missing values. The process is repeated iteratively until convergence.

For longitudinal data, in which observations are taken repeatedly over time and MAR assumptions are justifiable, several models are available that have reasonable performance relative to simple imputation methods. When the outcome variable is continuous, mixed-effect models for repeated measures (MMRM) can be used, with careful specification of the covariance matrix structure for the error term. For categorical responses and count data, the generalized linear mixed models (GLMM) have been proposed. The generalized estimating equations (GEE) approach is often used for longitudinal response data, but the method gives unbiased estimators if the missing-data mechanism only depends on the covariates included in the model (Fitzmaurice et al. 2000). Extensions of the approach are available, including the work by Robins et al. (1995) and Preisser et al. (2002), who proposed weighting schemes for GEE models that exhibit desirable performance under MAR assumptions.

There are many software programs designed to implement longitudinal data models under the ignorable situation. Commonly used examples include the R functions *lme* and *nlme* and the SAS procedures *MIXED, GLIMMIX, and NLMIXED*. However, caution should be exercised in the use of these models, since in the non-ignorable case the results will be subject to bias. In the following, we review some steps that should be taken in order to complement and strengthen the analyses based on these models.

2.3.4 Sensitivity Analyses

Once an analysis is performed based on a certain set of assumptions about the missing values, the results should be supported using appropriate sensitivity analyses that address the same research hypothesis. A key objective of the sensitivity analyses should be to evaluate how different assumptions influence the initial results that were obtained.

Although most primary analyses are performed under MAR assumptions, in general, it is not possible to rule out MNAR, and therefore the planned sensitivity analysis should include the scenario of MNAR. However, data analysis under MNAR assumptions is complex, and most of the common likelihood-based methods require specification of the joint distribution of the data and the missing data mechanism (Ibrahim and Molenberghs 2009). The approaches generally rely on maximum likelihood methods of estimation, based on mixed-effects models and normally distributed outcomes, and are intended to handle dropouts in clinical trials involving longitudinal data. Examples of the approaches for MNAR include selection models (Diggle and Kenward 1994), pattern-mixture models (Little and Wang 1996) and shared-parameter models (Little 1995; Kenward 1998). Shared-parameter models take into account the dependence between the measurement and the missingness processes, typically using random effects (Wu and Bailey 1989). On the other hand, both selection models and pattern-mixture models involve factoring the joint distribution of the full data and missing mechanism into suitable products of conditional distributions. For example, selection models are based on assumptions about the distribution of outcomes for all subjects and the distribution of missingness indicators conditional on the hypothetical complete outcomes. Pattern-mixture models, which are relatively more transparent and clinically interpretable, involve the conditional distribution of the data given the missingness pattern. In this case, when the number of patterns for the missing data is large relative to the sample size, there may be inadequate data to estimate parameters with reasonable degree of precisions. Thus, pattern-mixture models are not typically applied in situations with arbitrary missingness, but are generally restricted to cases with monotone missingness, where the number of patterns is manageable.

Tipping-point analyses are performed as an alternative approach to assess the robustness of study results corresponding to an assumed missingness mechanism. The approach essentially involves performing analyses with a range of values and searching the tipping point that reverses the study conclusion (e.g., from significant to non-significant). Since tipping-point analyses require exploring alternative model assumptions and values of the parameter, evaluation of the results may be cumbersome. To facilitate the interpretation of results from tipping-point analyses, alternative graphical displays have been proposed (see, e.g., Liublinska and Rubin 2014). The relatively transparent MNAR methods of pattern-mixture models and tipping-point analyses are practical sensitivity models to assess the robustness of the primary MAR results.

2.3.5 Estimands and Other Recent Regulatory Developments

Recently, the issue of missing values has been addressed in the context of the clinical question being asked and hence the quantity to be estimated, called estimand, and the nature of the sensitivity analyses that need to be performed. This was motivated by the aforementioned National Research

Council (NRC) report that addressed various aspects of missing data in clinical trials (NRC 2010). There have since been subsequent efforts involving diverse stakeholders to formulate a general framework to align trial objectives and planned inference (Akacha et al. 2017; ICH E9 (R1) 2017; LaVange and Permutt 2016).

The NRC report covered the underlying issues associated with missing data but did not give any recommendation about a specific method for handling them. However, it cautioned against the use of single imputation methods, such as LOCF mentioned earlier. The report emphasized the importance of sensitivity analyses, as well as the necessity of preventive steps that need to be taken at the design and conduct stages of a clinical trial. Some of the suggested measures include implementation of novel designs, other than the usual parallel group design; enhanced patient consent; encouraging patient compliance; and making greater efforts to collect post-discontinuation data.

As highlighted in the NCR report, the objective of an analysis strategy involving data with missing values should be to rule out bias in favor of the experimental drug that may have been introduced as a result of missing information or as a consequence of the action taken to handle the missing values. However, decision about the choice of the methods for the primary as well as sensitivity analyses is often complicated by various factors, including the lack of clarity about the intended objective, the actual target of inference, and the patient population to be included. As a result, this has led to the need to establish a framework based on the concept of estimands. In the following, we provide a high-level overview of the current thinking about estimands, while stressing the fact that the concept is still evolving and there are many issues that need to be addressed for effective implementation of the framework under discussion.

In a broad sense, an estimand is the quantity that is the target of inference in order to address the scientific question of interest posed by the trial objective (ICH E9 (R1) 2017). As such, it may be characterized by various attributes, including the population of interest, the variable (or endpoint), the handling of intercurrent or post-randomization events, and the summary statistics associated with the outcome variable.

The population of interest typically consists of the set of all study participants as defined by the protocol inclusion and exclusion criteria. This is referred to as the intent-to-treat (ITT) population. Usually, the ITT population is used to address the primary objective of establishing a treatment effect. However, there may be many valid scientific questions each requiring its own estimand, all of which may be used by regulatory agencies to assess the strength of the study results. In certain cases, the estimand may relate only to a subset of the randomized patients satisfying certain criteria, including any potential intercurrent or post-randomization events. In the literature this is often referred to as the "principal stratum." For example, the principal stratum may be the set of patients in which failure to adhere to treatment would not occur. In this case, the primary hypothesis relates to the treatment effect in this stratum. The variables used to characterize the estimand may be actual assessments taken during the study or functions of the measurements as well as intercurrent events. Finally, the population-level summary measure or statistic is a key component in the construction of the estimand and forms the basis for treatment effect comparisons.

Since intercurrent or post-randomization events can affect interpretation of results, there should be a clear specification of how they are incorporated in the construction of an estimand. Several strategies have been proposed to address intercurrent events, depending on the therapeutic and experimental contexts. In one approach, called treatment policy strategy, the value for the variable of interest is used without regard to the occurrence of intercurrent events. This approach is in alignment with the principle of ITT. However, in this strategy an estimand cannot be constructed with respect to a variable that cannot be measured after the intercurrent event. An alternative approach is the composite strategy, in which the intercurrent event is taken to be a component of the variable. For example, a responder may be defined in terms of a composite of no use of rescue medication and a favorable clinical outcome. In other situations, the estimand may be defined with respect to a principal stratum, which may be a subset of the study population that did not experience the intercurrent event. In contrast to the usual subgroup analysis, it is noted that principal stratification is defined based on a patient's potential post-randomization events. When the design involves repeated measurements, one may only focus on the responses observed prior to the occurrence of the intercurrent event. For example, in this case, also referred to as while-on-treatment strategy, if the goal is to assess treatment effect on a given symptom and a patient dies, one may only consider the effect on symptoms before death. Lastly, the strategy may involve defining a hypothetical scenario in which the intercurrent event would not occur and formulating the scientific question under the putative scenario. For example, in case a rescue medication is permitted in the protocol, the strategy requires assessing the outcome if no rescue medication was provided.

Underpinning the estimand framework is the importance of valid sensitivity analyses to assess the robustness of inferences from the main analysis. As discussed in the previous section, this should involve a number of analyses targeting the impact of deviations from some of the relevant underlying assumptions. The sensitivity analysis, as well as the estimand to which it is aligned, should be prespecified in the trial protocol.

The ongoing effort to develop a viable framework to bring the target of estimation, method of estimation, and sensitivity analysis in consonance with the objective of the trial can certainly lead to a better formulation of research hypothesis and interpretation of results and can facilitate collaboration among diverse stakeholders. In particular, it ensures alignment between pharmaceutical companies and regulatory agencies on expectations about trial design, data collection, and analytical strategies. However, as the concept evolves, further work may be needed to address operational issues that may arise in the course of the implementation of the framework.

2.3.6 Concluding Remarks

As elucidated in this section, one of the major threats to the validity of evidence from RCTs is the potential for bias associated with missing data. Despite the availability of regulatory guidelines and novel statistical approaches to address the issue, there is no silver bullet to solve the problem. Modern statistical analysis tools rely on untestable assumptions, and often require borrowing auxiliary information from experimental units with complete information. While sensitivity analyses are generally recommended as important tools to assess the degree to which results depend on model assumptions, the appropriateness of the approaches is heavily dependent on the extent of their coherence with the formulation of the original analysis. The only fullproof way to solve the missingness problem is not to have missing data. Although there are several proposed preventive steps that may be taken at the design and conduct stages of the trials to minimize their occurrence, in reality, missing values are unavoidable.

The recent efforts to define a framework in terms of estimands appears to be a step in the right direction, as that might help to enhance the communication between regulatory agencies and pharmaceutical companies by ensuring alignment early on in the process, as well as explicitly define the clinical question being addressed. From the broader perspective, the effort to harmonize the trial objectives with the analytical approaches and regulatory expectations may also contribute toward the overarching goal of improving the efficiency of the drug development paradigm. However, the concept is still evolving, and its refinement and successful implementation would undoubtedly require a gradual and iterative approach, involving inputs by all stakeholders.

2.4 NON-INFERIORITY STUDY

The distinguishing feature of a non-inferiority study is that the objective of the study is to show that the test treatment is not inferior to the control. A non-inferiority design can be employed in studies where the primary objective is either efficacy or safety. However, the design features and regulatory considerations are quite different for a study with a non-inferior efficacy objective and one with a non-inferiority safety objective. The non-inferiority design with an efficacy objective will be discussed first.

2.4.1 Efficacy Objective

The most direct way to establish the efficacy of a treatment is to show it to be superior to a placebo or an active agent in a superiority study. A placebo-controlled study is not always possible; therefore, use of an active control, where there is no expectation that the test drug is superior to the active control, may be necessary. The study objective is to show the test treatment is non-inferior to the active control within a protocol-specified non-inferiority margin (NIM). The rationale for a non-inferiority study primarily arises when the use of a placebo control is not ethical. The International Conference on Harmonization guidance E10: Choice of Control Group and Related Issues in Clinical Trials (ICH E10 2001) states that the use of placebo is unethical, "In cases where an available treatment is known to prevent serious harm, such as death or irreversible morbidity in the study population." Clearly, one does not need ICH E10 guidance to realize that withholding the available treatment is unethical. In some cases, such as oncology treatments, this ethical dilemma can be avoided by an add-on design in which the test drug or placebo is randomly added to the active treatment. However, often a direct comparison of the test drug to the active drug is called for, resulting in a non-inferiority study. A non-inferiority design may also be chosen for less critical considerations such as when randomization to placebo would make informed consent or enrollment problematic.

The critical value in a non-inferiority study is the NIM, i.e., what degree of inferiority must be ruled out in order to conclude non-inferiority of the test treatment to the control treatment. The manner in which the NIM is determined, its relationship to the non-inferior hypothesis, and its implications regarding study size and conclusions will be addressed next.

2.4.2 Non-inferiority Hypothesis / Non-inferiority Margin

In a superiority study the objective is to show that the test drug is superior to placebo or possibly an active control. In a hypothesis testing framework this implies,

$$H_0: T-P \leq 0 \text{ vs. } H_1: T-P > 0$$

where T and P represent the efficacy response for the test drug and placebo, respectively. In a non-inferiority study, the efficacy of the test drug is established indirectly by showing that it is not inferior to the active control (A) by more than a prespecified margin M (Figure 2.1). This implies a null and alternative hypothesis of

$$H_0: A-T \geq M \text{ vs. } H_1: A-T < M.$$

Clearly, the non-inferiority margin M is critical. If M is small then the demonstration of efficacy becomes very difficult resulting in a large sample size to reject inferiority. Likewise, if M is large then it may be incorrectly concluded that T is effective or, if effective, the difference between A and T may be clinically meaningful. This concept of clinically meaningful difference between A and T is an extra regulatory burden for non-inferiority studies as will be discussed in the following sections. Consequently, how

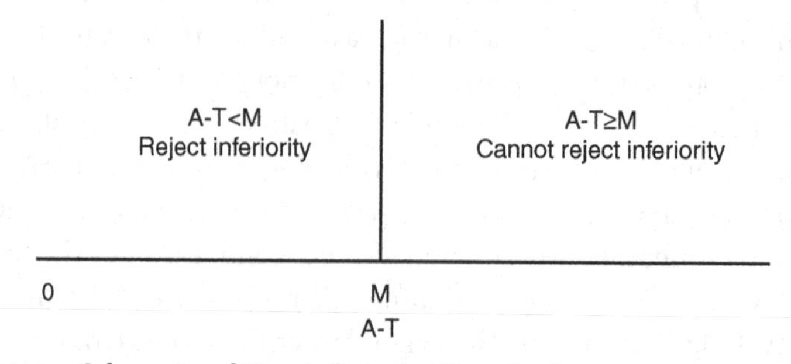

FIGURE 2.1 Schematic of Non-inferiority Hypothesis

M is determined and what it means to show that A-T is less than M are the critical aspects of a non-inferiority trial.

2.4.3 Determination of NIM

The determination of NIM, denoted as M above, requires clinical and statistical consideration, and is established based on the effect of the active control in past studies. This implies that in order to conduct a non-inferiority study there must be a suitable active control whose efficacy has been reliably established in previous studies. The NIM is usually not the point estimate of the active treatment effect in the previous studies, but rather, the effect of the active control, conservatively defined as the limit of the confidence interval closest to the null; e.g., a lower confidence bound (LCB) (typically 97.5% or 95%, one sided) of the mean effect of the active control in the previous studies. This value is acceptable to regulators because it gives a degree of confidence that the active treatment effect would be at least this large (compared to the non-observed placebo) in the non-inferiority study. The conservative nature of this method of determining the NIM should be stressed. If the LCB is close to 0 due to variability of the estimate of the active treatment effect, then a non-inferiority study to show efficacy of the test agent is not feasible. The concept mentioned earlier of a clinically meaningful difference between the test and the active control, which implies the need to preserve a given proportion of the efficacy of the active control is an added conservative burden imposed on many non-inferiority studies. It is beneficial and useful to discuss these concepts in the context of a real example. This example is given in the FDA Guidance Document on non-inferiority studies (FDA 2016).

2.4.4 Example: FDA Guidance Document

This example concerns the use of a non-inferiority study for approval of a new thrombolytic agent for the treatment of acute myocardial infarction. Streptokinase was the active comparator and its effect was established by a meta-analysis of placebo-controlled trials. Streptokinase yielded a 2.6% benefit in mortality compared to placebo with a one-sided 95% lower bound of 2.1%. The one-sided 95% lower confidence bound of 2.1% was taken as the effect of streptokinase for the purposes of the NI study rather than the most likely estimate of 2.6% because the NI study is dependent on something that is not measured in the NI study, namely, the effect of streptokinase over placebo. Thus, the conservative estimate of 2.1% was

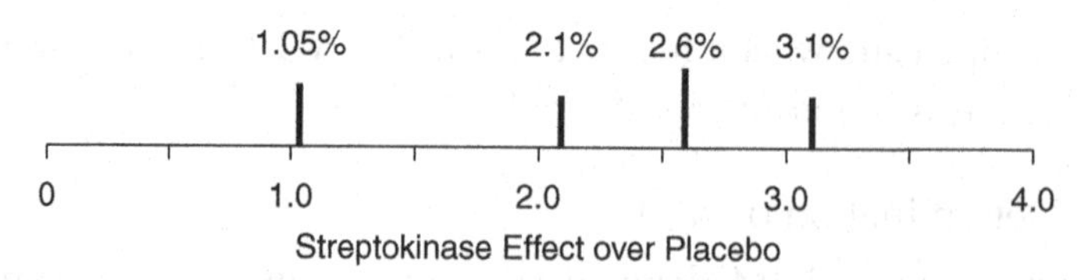

FIGURE 2.2 Effect of Streptokinase on Mortality Compared to Placebo

selected to increase the confidence that this effect would be present in the NI study. While 2.1% could serve as an acceptable NIM to show efficacy for the new agent, the clinical /regulatory decision was made that the NI study should rule out a loss of more than half of the benefit of streptokinase to be an acceptable alternative. The NI study would therefore have to rule out an NIM of a 1.05% increase in mortality in patients treated with the new thrombolytic drug compared to those treated with streptokinase. Figure 2.2 illustrates these values.

To rule out an increase in mortality of 1.05%, a one-sided 97.5% upper confidence bound of the test drug minus streptokinase difference in mortality must be below 1.05%.

2.4.5 Implications of Choice of NIM

As indicated above, there are stringent criteria for a successful NI study. An NI study with an NIM intending to preserve half of the effect of the active drug requires approximately four times the number of subjects of an NI study intending to show the test drug is simply better than placebo. In the above example, this is an NIM of 1.05% compared to an NIM of 2.1%. It should also be noted that this 95% lower confidence limit of 2.1% is a conservative estimate of the streptokinase effect.

An NI study designed to rule out the loss of a proportion of the active comparator benefit implies a "comparative effectiveness" standard that is not included in the Federal Food, Drug, and Cosmetic Act. As a result, the following statement was placed in the Federal Register of August 1, 1995 (60 FR 39180 at 39181), as an FDA position by then FDA's Deputy Commissioner for Policy, William Schultz: "In certain circumstances, however, it may be important to consider whether a new product is less effective than available alternative therapies." The two circumstances given are: 1. Disease is life-threatening or capable of causing irreversible morbidity (e.g., stroke or heart attack); 2. Disease is a contagious illness that poses serious consequences to the health of others.

Thus, the ethical reasons for the use of an active control and an NI study is the same as the ethical reason to assure the test drug maintains a proportion of the active control's effect. In the streptokinase example, the 95% lower confidence bound of 2.1% would not be acceptable because it does not assure any proportion of the streptokinase effect preserved in the NI study. Preserving 50% of the effect was selected as the NIM. However, if an NI design is used when the ethical imperatives do not apply, such as when randomization to placebo would make informed consent or enrollment problematic, then according to the Act and the 1995 wording, the study should not have to show that the test drug maintains a proportion of the effect of the active control, and the 95% lower confidence limit should be acceptable as the NIM.

2.4.6 Strength of a Non-inferiority Study

The regulatory strength of a non-inferiority study depends on three critical conditions. Absence of any one of these three conditions would not allow an efficacy inference for the test drug. First, there must be reliable information about the effect the active control drug had in past studies compared to placebo. A consistent positive effect of the active control is required to establish the NIM. Treatment in diseases where an active drug does not consistently show a benefit over placebo, e.g., major depression, would not allow for establishing an NIM and consequently would not be a candidate for an NI Study. In the above setting, this may be overcome by the 95% lower confidence limit using the A-P historical estimate, but in the case where previous studies do not show a consistent effect over placebo, it is recommended to discuss the design with the regulators. In determining the NIM, study-to-study variability in the estimate of the active control effect must be taken into account in forming the NIM. This implies a random-effects meta-analysis of the existing studies to estimate the mean effect of the active drug and the lower confidence limit of the mean. If the efficacy of the active control has been established in only one study, then a higher degree of confidence on the lower limit may be required.

The second condition is that the effect the active control drug has in the current NI study is similar to the effect observed in past studies. The validity of an NI study is dependent on assuming something that is not measured in the study, namely, that the active control had its expected effect in the NI study. This is sometimes referred to as the constancy assumption. This is somewhat addressed by using the lower confidence bound as the estimate of the active treatment effect that leads to high confidence that the effect of the active control is at least as strong in the NI study. In order to strengthen the constancy assumption, there should be similarity between the important characteristics of the current NI study with those of prior studies that established the efficacy of the active compound.

The third condition is that the NI study reliably estimates the effect of the test drug relative to the active control. This is predominately relating to the quality of the conduct of the NI study. Almost all departures from "quality" lead to a reduction in the estimate of the active minus test effect. In a superiority study this reduction is toward the null hypothesis. However, in a non-inferiority study this reduction is toward the alternative hypothesis and, hence, makes it more likely to reject the null and conclude non-inferiority. Thus, discontinuations from treatment, missing data, adherence to treatment, all tend to reduce treatment differences and, therefore, need to be assessed before concluding non-inferiority of the test drug to the control. Due to its conservative estimate of the treatment difference, the ITT analysis alone is often not considered sufficient by regulators to conclude non-inferiority and, hence, the on-treatment analysis, even with potential bias, is important as a sensitivity analysis in an NI trial.

2.4.7 Synthesis Method for Non-inferiority

Non-inferiority may be established by a direct comparison of the results from the studies used to estimate the effect of the active control with the results of the NI Study (sometimes referred to as the synthesis method). When the parameter of interest is the mean, the effect of the active control compared to placebo is estimated from the existing studies by the contrast of means A-P with variance V_1 and the effect of the active control compared to the test drug from the NI Study by the contrast of means A-T with variance V_2. The combined contrast of (A-P)-(A-T) yields an indirect estimate of the effect of the test drug compared to placebo (T-P) with variance $V_1 + V_2$. The lower confidence bound on this indirect estimate of A-T being greater than 0 establishes the efficacy of T. The lower confidence bound by the synthesis method, e.g., one sided 95% confidence interval (CI), (A-T) – 1.645 $(V_1 + V_2)^{0.5}$, is always greater than the lower confidence bound by method 1, (A-T) – 1.645 $(V_1^{0.5} + V_2^{0.5})$ and, hence, the proportion of the effect of A preserved by T is greater. Accordingly, one is more likely to conclude non-inferiority by the synthesis method. It should be noted that all of the discussion above relating to the first method apply to the synthesis method as well and, in particular, the assumption of a constant effect of the control A in the previous studies and the NI study.

2.4.8 Summary Points

- Superiority studies are preferable to an active-controlled NI Study.
- NI studies are necessary when available treatment is known to prevent serious harm, such as death or irreversible morbidity.
- A consistent effect shown by the active control in past studies is a necessary basis for an NI study and the effect of the active control is conservatively estimated by a lower confidence limit.
- A constancy of effect of the active treatment from past studies to the current NI study is a necessary assumption.
- The NIM is a crucial aspect of an NI study. This margin is often smaller than the effect of the active control in order to assure that a given proportion of the effect of the active control is preserved by the test drug.
- Similarity of important characteristics of the NI study and the past studies used to establish the effect of the active control, as well as the quality of the conduct of the NI study are important regulatory review criteria.

2.4.9 Non-inferiority Study with a Safety Objective

Statistical and regulatory considerations regarding non-inferiority studies with a safety objective are somewhat different from those discussed for an efficacy objective. These arise primarily around the determination of the NIM and related issues. Non-inferiority studies designed to show efficacy of the test drug require an NIM based on the effect of the active control in past studies. This implies that the active control is consistently and reliably effective in past studies. Without the NIM, efficacy cannot be inferred from a non-inferiority study. A frequently occurring regulatory setting for a non-inferiority safety study begins with a suspected safety issue regarding serious, low-incidence adverse events of a marketed drug, e.g., the association of cardiovascular events with nonsteroidal anti-inflammatory drugs, particularly Cox-2 inhibitors. A regulatory body may mandate a study to address the concern. The study may be either active or placebo-controlled with the objective to show that the test drug does not have a "clinically unacceptable" higher incidence of the adverse experience (AE) compared to the control. Typically, the actual incidence of the AE in the control group may be difficult to estimate. Thus, the NIM in an efficacy study, from which effectiveness can be inferred, is quite different from an NIM in a safety study, from which only an agreed-upon level of excess risk can be ruled out. The concept of "clinically unacceptable" is ambiguous and subjective in application and consequently, while the NIM in a safety study should be determined in a clinically rigorous way, it is less objective than in efficacy studies. In addition, in order that any excess risk of a serious AE is acceptable, there must be some benefit that leads to the NIM being based on a risk–benefit assessment. However, safety studies can be conducted without establishing an NIM and can be useful for regulatory purposes, e.g., the Evaluating Adverse Events in a Global Smoking Cessation Study (EAGLES) of varenicline and serious neuropsychiatric adverse events (Anthenelli 2016). This raises the general question, what then is the purpose of an NIM in a safety study.

The need for an NIM and the consequences of including an NIM or not in a safety study should be considered in the regulatory context of the safety issue. Prospective Randomized Evaluation of Celecoxib Integrated Safety vs. Ibuprofen or Naproxen (PRECISION) (Nissen 2016; Gaffney 2016) was a regulatory-mandated, large non-inferiority safety study to assess whether a Cox-2 nonsteroidal anti-inflammatory drug increased the rate of cardiovascular adverse events compared to two traditional nonsteroidal anti-inflammatory drugs (NSAIDs). An NIM was used in PRECISION. Some rigor can be introduced by defining the NIM to be the level of increased risk that would be "clinically unacceptable" in the context of the "level of benefit" that is provided by the treatment. The PRECISION study NIM of 1.33 was determined by considering a potential benefit of Cox-2 on serious gastrointestinal events in conjunction with a clinically acceptable excess risk based on the expected cardiovascular event rate in the NSAID control group. Even when the NIM is determined by a clinical/scientific method, it is still subjective. The NIM in a non-inferiority safety study does not have the data-determined objectivity that the NIM in a non-inferiority efficacy study has. However, the NIM is a strong determinant of study size and, consequently, the cost and time necessary to ensure the reliability of the study results. For example, the sample size needed with an NIM of 1.33 is about 37% larger than the sample size needed with an NIM of 1.40. Thus, when an NIM can be determined by a strong clinical method and agreed upon with the regulatory body, it provides important scientific context for the design, conduct, and analysis of the study and serves the purpose of ruling out a predefined unacceptable increase in risk. It also serves as an objective regulatory criterion that the study results have or have not ruled out an unacceptable increase in risk.

In contrast to PRECISION, the EAGLES study (Anthenelli 2016, Gaffney 2016) was designed without an NIM. EAGLES was also a regulatory-mandated, large safety study to assess whether varenicline had an increased rate of serious neuropsychiatric adverse events compared to placebo and two other methods of smoking cessation. For many reasons it was not feasible to determine an NIM by a strong clinical rationale. Without an NIM there is no study hypothesis. Consequently, the objective of EAGLES was to estimate the rate differences and the uncertainty around these estimates. Sample size was determined, with agreement with the regulators, by a prespecified width of the 95% confidence interval in estimating the rate differences in neuropsychiatric adverse events. However, with no agreed-upon unacceptable level of increased risk to rule out, the interpretation of EAGLES is more difficult from a regulatory perspective.

The use of the 95% CI to determine study size does not necessarily lead to smaller trials than NIM-based trials, or other trials that use less rigorous approaches. There is a one-to-one correspondence between the width of the confidence interval and an NIM. However, the use of the 95% CI to determine study size may lead to a better understanding of the uncertainty around risk estimation and the cost to reduce the uncertainty, which may in turn lead to smaller trials. For example, as stated above, the sample size needed with an NIM of 1.33 is about 37% larger than the sample size needed with an NIM of 1.40. However, the upper confidence interval of the point estimate of the observed hazard ratio (HR) is reduced from 1.226HR to only 1.190HR by this increase in study size. This reduction in uncertainty can be assessed relative to the increase in study cost, study duration, and time to clinical knowledge of the study results.

2.4.10 Summary Points

- The NIM in a non-inferiority safety study does not have the data-determined objectivity of an NIM in a non-inferiority efficacy study. While the NIM in a safety study should be determined in a clinically rigorous way, it is more subjective than the NIM in efficacy studies.
- Additional rigor can be introduced in the safety NI study by defining the NIM to be the level of increased risk that would be "clinically unacceptable" in the context of the "level of benefit" of the treatment.

- When an NIM can be determined with a strong clinical rationale, it serves as an objective regulatory criterion that the study results have or have not ruled out an unacceptable increase in risk.
- When an NIM cannot be determined by a strong clinical rationale, a safety study can be sized by the width of the 95% CI.
- The use of the width of the 95% CI to determine study size may lead to a better understanding of the uncertainty around risk estimation and the cost of reducing uncertainty and thereby lead to smaller trials.

2.5 INNOVATIVE TRIAL DESIGNS

Novel and nonstandard study designs are promoted both by pharmaceutical companies and regulatory agencies to streamline the current drug development and regulatory approval processes. This is especially given heightened attention in research concerning rare diseases, oncology, and other areas with unmet medical needs. However, these designs are inherently complex, and are associated with important statistical and operational issues that require careful considerations. Notably, a recent guidance document from the US FDA (2018a) highlights four requirements for successful implementation of an adaptive design: controlling the chance of erroneous conclusions, reliable estimation of treatment effects, prespecification of relevant details of the design, and safeguarding trial integrity. Next, we give a summary of a few of the commonly used novel approaches, including adaptive and flexible designs, enrichment studies, and studies conducted under the so-called master protocols.

2.5.1 Adaptive Designs

Adaptive designs permit modifications to various attributes of the trial based on analysis of data from subjects in the study, while ensuring that the integrity of the trial is not compromised. The modification may involve study procedures, including eligibility criteria, dose levels and duration of treatment; sample size; or statistical methods. Examples of adaptive design methods include adaptive randomization, group sequential designs, sample size reestimation, adaptive dose-finding designs, as well as adaptive-seamless Phase II/III trial designs (Chow et al. 2005).

2.5.2 Adaptive Randomization

In comparative trials, assignment of study subjects to treatment groups may be adjusted either based on baseline characteristics (*covariate-adaptive treatment assignment*) or comparative outcome data. The former is conducted with a view to achieving balance between treatment groups with respect to important baseline covariates. An example is the so-called minimization approach, proposed by Pocock and Simon (1975), in which consecutive patients are systematically allocated to treatments so as to minimize any difference on the selected prognostic factors.

In response-adaptive randomization, the principal goal is to increase the probability of success by modifying the randomization schedule as a function of observed treatment effect. An example is the *randomized play-the-winner rule*, which uses an urn model for patient allocation (Rosenberger 1999). An appealing feature of response-adaptive randomization is that, on average, the more efficacious treatment arm will be studied on a higher proportion of study subjects. In addition, there are also situations where the approach may lead to efficient statistical procedures, including reduced variability of treatment effect estimates. The assignment probability (π_a) may be determined using alternative approaches. One method due to Thall and Wathen (2007) computes the probability as:

$$\pi_a = \frac{[P(T>C)]^r}{\left[P(T>C)\right]^r + \left[1-P(T>C)\right]^r}$$

where r is a positive tuning parameter, and $P(T > C)$ is the posterior probability that the new agent (T) is better than the control (C), based on accumulated data, and using the uniform prior distribution.

Adaptive randomization strategies may not be advisable in all situations. In fact, the added complexity, in terms of execution, analysis, and interpretation, may not justify their use relative to standard trial designs. In particular, their application in Phase III studies may require caution due to the potential for bias arising from time trends associated with any prognostic factors. In such cases, block randomization and stratified analysis approaches are recommended. Korn and Freidlin (2011) provide a discussion of the pros and cons of adaptive randomization.

2.5.3 Sample Size Reestimation

In some situations, there may initially be inadequate information about certain parameters involved in sample size determination to achieve the desired power and Type I error rates. Examples of such parameters include the detectable effect size, measures of dispersion, or the null response rate in the comparison of two proportions. Study size, therefore, may be adjusted based on appropriately defined sample size reestimation techniques using data observed during an interim period.

One of the earliest approaches proposed by Wittes and Brittain (1990) uses an internal pilot study. More specifically, the trial is designed using an initial estimate of the parameter of interest. An interim analysis is then performed to estimate the parameter, which in turn is used to recalculate the sample size. This approach typically results in small inflation of the Type I error rate, which may be substantial when the interim analysis is based on very few observations.

When there is uncertainty about the effect size, several strategies may be followed to achieve the desired result. An adaptive approach, often called unblinded sample size reestimation, consists in starting with a modest sample size, and then increasing the size, following an interim comparative analysis. This approach has known shortcomings. First, a large sample size may lead to detection of clinically irrelevant effects. In addition, inadvertent dissemination of interim results may compromise the integrity of the conduct and reporting of the trial (Mauer et al. 2012). Further, without proper adjustment, such an approach can inflate the Type I error probability (Proschan and Hunsberger 1995).

To control the Type I error rate, combination tests have been proposed, using the *p*-values computed at the different stages of the trial. Specifically, let P_1 and P_2 be the *p*-values associated, respectively, with the test of the null hypothesis at the interim look and then at the end of the trial based on the reestimated sample size. Bauer and Kohne (1994) propose a test defined on the product, $T = P_1P_2$, which has a $\exp(\chi^2_4/2)$ distribution under the null. One may also construct a test statistic using the inverse normal cumulative distribution transformation:

$$Z = w_1Z_1 + w_2Z_2$$

where $Z_i = \Phi^{-1}(1 - P_i)$, and the w_i $(i = 1, 2)$ are prespecified weights such that $w_1^2 + w_2^2 = 1$. Under the null, Z has a $N(0,1)$ distribution. See also Cui et al. (1999) and Denne (2001), among others, for related approaches.

It may be noted that approaches based on prespecified weights are often criticized on the ground that they violate the sufficiency principle, and hence may not be efficient. Further, their dependence on nonstandard tests and *p*-values make them less attractive. A more appealing strategy involves the group sequential approach, in which the trial is designed with maximum sample size, and then interim analyses are performed with the goal of stopping the trial for efficacy or futility or adjusting the sample size. Notably, Mehta and Pocock (2011) proposed the promising-zone approach in which the sample size is increased when interim results appear to be promising. More specifically, at the interim analysis, the promising zone can be characterized with respect to the estimated conditional power (CP), i.e., the probability of statistically significant result at the end of the trial, given the observed data, and assuming no change in the observed treatment effect and planned sample size. Using the estimated CP, the interim outcome may then be classified into unfavorable, favorable, or promising zones. If the interim result falls in the promising zone, the sample size may be increased, assuming plausible values for any relevant parameters; otherwise, there will be no change to the design. The approach is appealing because of its ease of implementation, since conventional final inference can be performed without inflating the overall Type I error. Indeed, Chen et al. (2004) argue that with CP >0.5, one can increase the sample size and use conventional test statistics while preserving the Type I error. However, it has been shown by Gaffney and Ware (2017) that the conventional statistic compared to the standard critical value (e.g., $Z - 1.96$ for $\alpha = 0.05$) will be conservative.

In the above discussion, while the focus has been on preserving the Type I error, it should also be noted that determination of a valid point estimate and confidence intervals following sample size reestimation may not be straightforward. This is, in fact, an issue of regulatory and methodological importance associated with all adaptive designs, requiring caution in the reporting of the accompanying study results (Wassmer and Brannath 2016).

2.5.4 Sequential Designs

Sequential designs are applied in situations where the objective consists in early termination of a trial, either for futility or overwhelming efficacy. In planning such trials, it is critical to specify the purpose, frequency of analysis, and procedures to be applied to control Type I error probabilities. Some of the strategies require prospective definitions of both the number of interim analyses and the amount of information to be observed. The choice of a particular strategy also depends on the intended purpose and operational considerations. For example, the O'Brien–Fleming approach tends to require strong evidence for early stopping (O'Brien and Fleming 1979); while Pocock's method tends to lead to more frequent early stopping

(Pocock 1977). On the other hand, the general alpha-spending approach provides flexibility about the number and timing of interim looks, since it mainly depends on specification of a function for how the Type I error probability is spent (Lan and DeMets 1983). However, even this approach may result in inflation of Type I error if the timing of interim analysis is based on knowledge of the observed treatment effects.

As mentioned earlier, when using group sequential designs, estimates of treatment effects are known to be biased, and confidence intervals do not have the desired nominal levels. Therefore, appropriate adjustment should be made to the estimates when reporting such results (Jennison and Turnbull 1999; Wassmer and Brannath 2016). Further, independent monitoring of the study is essential to safeguard the integrity of the trial and credibility of the results (see, e.g., Ellenberg et al. 2002).

Group sequential designs may be more efficient than sample-size reestimation designs; however, depending on the circumstances, sample-size reestimation could still be the preferred design (Levin et al. 2013). The choice of the sequential design may depend on the stage of development and prior knowledge and expectation of the treatment effect.

2.5.5 Adaptive Designs for Dose and Treatment Selection

Modifications could also be made to treatment arms, including doses of the same agent, based on interim results. In early-phase trials, adaptive dose-ranging trials may be conducted to select an optimal dose or doses for further evaluation. An example is the Continual Reassessment Method (CRM), a model-based approach discussed in Chapter 1, which involves fitting a dose-toxicity curve to estimate the maximum tolerated dose for a new drug (Le Tourneau et al. 2009).

In late-phase drug development, an adaptive dose-modification design may allow interim selection of candidate doses from two or more competing candidates, thereby permitting assignment of future patients to the selected treatment arms. Seamless Phase II/III trials are sometimes used as a viable option when there is interest to shorten time-to-market of a new medicine, by addressing two objectives in the same study; namely, dose selection, at an interim analysis, and efficacy determination, at the end of the study. In such designs, suitable procedures should be used to pool information from patients enrolled before and after the adaptation to perform inference at the final analysis, while controlling the Type I error. Examples of approaches include the combination test techniques described earlier, or the adaptive Dunnett design (see, e.g., Stallard and Todd 2010).

In general, the choice of a specific approach requires a careful evaluation of several factors, including trial objective, outcome measure, and other therapeutic and practical considerations.

2.5.6 Adaptive Enrichment Designs

Adaptive enrichment designs allow modifications to the patient population based on comparative interim results. The final analysis may involve multiple hypotheses; thereby requiring appropriate procedures to adjust for multiplicity (see, e.g., Wassmer and Brannath 2016).

Enrichment designs have especially become an attractive option in oncology, as the focus of drug development shifted from those centered on cytotoxic agents (i.e., those agents that may stop cancer cells from dividing and growing or cause tumors to shrink) to those using molecularly targeted agents (which target specific molecular markers) or use a patient's immune response to attack cancer cells. To implement such designs, it is essential to ensure that the molecular marker is well established (i.e., is strongly correlated with the outcome measure) and that a diagnostic tool for evaluating it is available. Further, it should be ascertained that the study drug is not effective in the marker-negative patients. If the latter is not known, the randomization should be stratified by molecular marker positivity or negativity or use more complex designs with a common protocol (Simon 2017a). When enrichment designs are used in seamless Phase II/III trials, the required sample size and analysis for each phase may be evaluated using the same or different endpoints. For example, assuming progression-free survival for end of Phase II and overall survival for Phase III, the corresponding analyses may be performed after the following numbers of events E_p (p = I or II) have been observed:

$$E_p = 4\left(\frac{Z_{1-\alpha_p} + Z_{\beta_p}}{\log \nabla_p}\right)$$

where two-sided significance level α and higher power $1-\beta$ are typically used for Phase III, for detecting the respective hazard ratio ∇p (Schoenfeld 1983).

2.5.7 Master Protocols

Recently, more complex designs have been proposed to allow treatment arm selection or subgroup identification adaptively using a common protocol.

For example, as stated in a recent US FDA guideline (US FDA 2018b), first-in-human multiple expansion-cohort trials involving oncology drugs and biologics may be conducted using a single protocol to address several cohort-specific objectives, starting with an initial dose-escalation phase, and including additional cohorts to evaluate different aspects of the drug. The latter may include assessment of safety or efficacy in specific populations or evaluation of the predictive value of a potential biomarker. To minimize the accompanying risks to patients with such trials, it is important to restrict the approach to patients with unmet needs, and also to have adequate infrastructure to ensure that emerging results and safety signals are communicated in real time to regulators and other stakeholders.

More generally, master protocols may be developed with the intent of designing and conducting clinical trials that address multiple objectives simultaneously. This may include the evaluation of more than one investigational drug or more than one cancer type within the same protocol. A master protocol may be based on a fixed or adaptive design, but it is generally considered after the recommended Phase II dose (RP2D) has been established in an adult patient population. While there are alternative designs used in master protocols, it is noted that there is a lack of consistency in the definitions of the terms for the studies. Common examples, discussed below, are the so-called basket trials, umbrella trials, and platform trials.

2.5.7.1 Basket Trials

In a basket trial, a master protocol may be developed to evaluate a treatment regimen in different subpopulations, each with a specific objective and scientific rationale (Figure 2.3). The subpopulations are generally defined by various demographic characteristics, biomarkers, or disease attributes, including tumor type, number of prior therapies, or disease stage. Basket trials are exploratory in nature, and the substudies often involve a single arm. In oncology, one often aims at estimating the overall response rate (ORR) as a measure of drug activity in the various subpopulations, since survival endpoints are not feasible in such designs. Hence, the planned sample size may be calculated to rule out a clinically trivial response rate as determined by the lower bound of a 95% confidence interval.

To limit exposure to an ineffective drug, basket trials typically employ designs such as the approach proposed by Simon (1989). The response rate may be estimated both for the subpopulations as well as for the pooled data. Cunanan et al. (2017) suggest an enhanced approach in which an

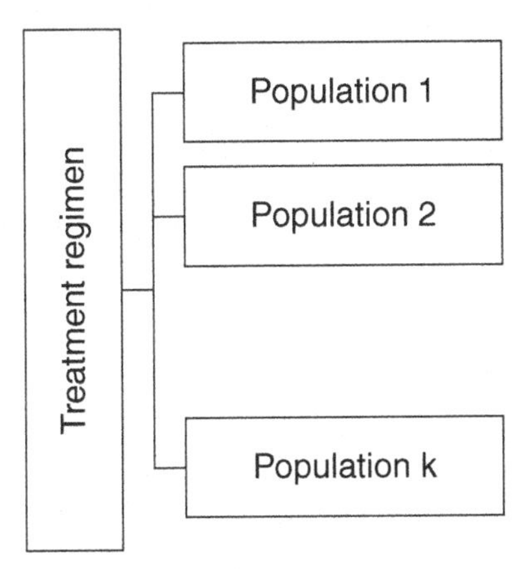

FIGURE 2.3 Schematic Representation of a Master Protocol with Basket Trial Design

interim analysis is first performed to rule out homogeneity of the response rates across subpopulations. If there is evidence of heterogeneity, then separate two-stage designs are conducted for each subpopulation; otherwise the usual two-stage design is performed on the pooled data.

Statistical approaches are also available that permit borrowing information across subpopulations. LeBlanc et al. (2009) propose a frequentist method, while others advocate Bayesian hierarchical modeling to implement information borrowing. One approach, due to Thall et al. (2003), allows treatment effects to differ across subpopulations, while assuming the effects are exchangeable and correlated. According to Berry et al. (2013), the Bayesian hierarchical model seems to have lower overall Type I error rate compared to Bayesian or frequentist approaches applied to each subpopulation. The power may, however, be low in situations where the drug is inactive in most strata. Also, the performance of the approach may be questionable if there is inadequate information on the outcome due to small sample size, which typically is the case in Phase II trials (Freidlin and Korn 2013).

Simon et al. (2016) introduced a Bayesian design that requires prespecification of stratum-specific prior probabilities under two scenarios: homogeneous and heterogeneous responses across subpopulations. More specifically, a quantity λ is specified as the prior for homogeneity, and another prior γ for a hypothesized response rate π_1, considered acceptable activity. The approach can readily be implemented using accessible software.

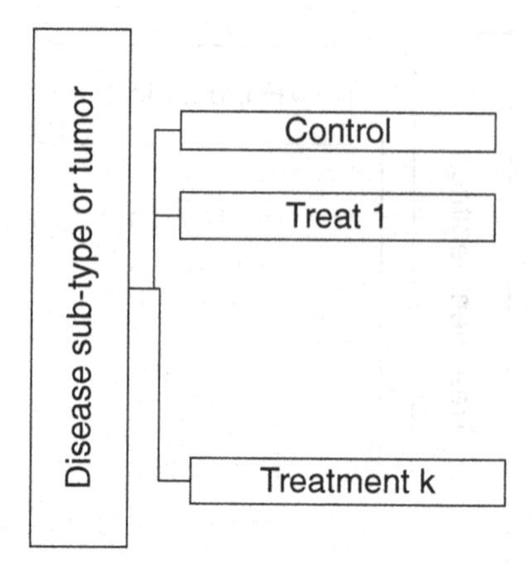

FIGURE 2.4 Schematic Representation of a Master Protocol with Umbrella Trial Design

Some authors have proposed a hybrid approach in which a Bayesian hierarchical model is used in the final stage if homogeneity of effect across subpopulations is established at the interim analysis (Liu et al. 2017). For basket trials, Yuan et al. (2016) and Chen et al. (2016) propose procedures that ensure control of the family-wise error rate through pruning of subpopulations.

2.5.7.2 Umbrella Trials

When there is interest to assess multiple treatment regimens in a single-disease population, umbrella trials may be conducted using a common protocol (Figure 2.4). Typically, such trials use randomized controlled designs, where the control may be the standard of care (SOC) for all substudies.

2.5.7.3 Platform Trials

In oncology, Simon (2017a) defines a platform trial as a single-histology randomized Phase II study in which multiple biomarkers and multiple drugs are studied. A key feature of such a design is that there is no prior assumption about which treatment is appropriate for a subpopulation; instead treatments are randomized to biomarker strata. The randomization may be performed adaptively, with the randomization given greater weights in favor of subpopulations with relatively higher response rates in the course of the study.

Treatment effects in platform studies may be analyzed using Bayesian hierarchical models. However, as noted in Simon (2017a), the approach may not control the Type I error rate in the conventional sense and may also suffer from prognostic imbalances as a result of the adaptive randomization. Hobbs et al. (2016) propose a framework for trials with binary endpoints using Bayesian modeling and adaptive randomization. The framework allows dropping poorly performing agents, incorporating new candidate agents, and controlling for multiplicity. In a recent paper, Kaizer et al. (2018) introduce a related approach with desirable power properties.

Frequentist approaches, although not common, are also available. A main technical issue is the computational burden associated with the extension of two-arm group sequential designs to platform and related trials, while guaranteeing strong control of the Type1 error rate. Ghosh et al. (2017) provide an efficient algorithm that can compute decision boundaries for adaptive designs involving multiple comparisons over multiple stages.

2.5.7.4 Regulatory and Operational Considerations with Novel Trials

Whether the goal is to implement adaptive randomization, sample size reestimation, seamless Phase II/III trial design, or a master protocol, the implementation of the approaches requires application of sound statistical methods and principles, and well-established operational processes. For example, while a master protocol undoubtedly has the potential to enhance efficiency, it is inherently complex, and hence requires extra effort to ensure patient safety and quality data that is acceptable to regulators. In fact, without proper measures to mitigate the associated operational and analytical challenges, the trials may not only increase the risk to patients but can also cause unnecessary delay in the approval of a potentially beneficial treatment option.

Operationally, basket trials may be less challenging than those using umbrella designs, since the former is conducted by a single sponsor. However, when biomarkers are used to define subpopulations, the process of assigning individuals with multiple biomarkers to a subpopulation will need clear justification.

It is always advisable to prespecify all the intended modifications and adaptations that will take place after the trial is initiated (see, e.g., US FDA 2018a). Especially in confirmatory trials, careful attention should be paid to Type I error inflation, bias associated with treatment effect estimate, as well as potential heterogeneity of the patient population induced by the modifications of trial procedures (Chow et al. 2005). One major problem with adaptive designs is the issue of multiplicity. In master protocols, for example, frequentist inference corresponding to the various study groups can potentially lead to false positive findings. Therefore, appropriate adjustment should be made to ensure preservation of Type I error and reliability of point and interval estimates.

From the standpoint of safety reporting, the issues include the difficulty in the prompt identification of adverse events, in the face of the rapid enrollment of study subjects in the various substudies or study stages. Therefore, these designs require the establishment of independent data monitoring committees, to ensure real-time review of serious adverse events, and to make decisions regarding study modification or termination.

Bayesian adaptive designs are frequently used in informing decision-making, at times borrowing information from external sources for informative priors. In such cases, controlling Type I error probability at a conventional level may eliminate the benefits of borrowing. In practice, although the Bayesian approach is used for study design and computing probabilities, regulatory requirements relating to Type I and Type II error must be satisfied using extensive simulation. As highlighted in a recent FDA guideline, "any clinical trial whose design is governed by Type I error probability and power considerations is inherently a frequentist trial, regardless of whether Bayesian methods are used in the trial design or analysis" (US FDA 2018a).

In summary, with any complex adaptive or other novel designs, it is prudent to have early discussion with the appropriate regulatory bodies to ensure alignment on the intended strategy. To facilitate the effectiveness of the FDA evaluation of such designs, sponsors should provide adequate documentation, including design selection rationale, adaptation strategy, roles of data monitoring groups, prespecified statistical methods, and details of any simulation experiments (see, e.g., US FDA 2018b). Finally, it is important to note that, regardless of trial design, regulators still require substantial evidence of efficacy and safety in a well-defined patient population for approval. Thus, in most cases, it is not surprising to see trials being conducted using a conventional design at the confirmatory stage.

2.6 BAYESIAN ANALYSIS IN A REGULATORY FRAMEWORK

2.6.1 Introduction

As mentioned elsewhere in this monograph, the importance of Bayesian statistical methods in drug development has garnered increased attention in recent years, thanks in part to the role they play in areas where application of frequentist approaches may be challenging or may not be as effective. In the frequentist paradigm, historical information is generally considered informally, and even then, only at the design stage, such as when performing sample size determination or study subject selection and recruitment. In contrast, a major appeal of Bayesian techniques is that they enhance decision-making not only at the design stage of a trial, but also during the conduct and analysis phases. The techniques are especially suited in trials involving adaptive and other flexible designs in which historical or accumulating evidence can be leveraged to modify certain aspects of the trials, with a view to accelerating the process of generating evidence relative to the risks and benefits of a new agent.

A central concept of both the frequentist and Bayesian approaches is the likelihood principle, which states that the likelihood function contains all the information generated by an experiment about a parameter of interest. In a typical inference problem, the frequentist perspective is hypothesis testing of a claim about the null parameter and an acceptance or rejection of the claim based on the observed data only. The frequentist approach is concerned with the likelihood of the data given the parameter, whereas the Bayesian approach is concerned with the likelihood of the parameter given the data. In the Bayesian framework, previous data or even subjective considerations are used to form a prior distribution of the parameter. The likelihood function from the experimental observations is used to update the prior distribution of a parameter, resulting in the posterior distribution. As such, Bayesian conclusions are drawn only based on the posterior distribution. An important quantity obtained from a posterior distribution is the predictive probability, i.e., the conditional chance of an unobserved outcome, such as a trial being successful, or a clinical outcome being positive, given the observed data. Bayesian decisions are often made with respect to the magnitude of the posterior probability. For example, a Bayesian hypothesis testing problem may be formulated in terms of the conditional probability that a specific claim is true, given the observed data.

Historically, two major constraints have limited the wide use of Bayesian statistical techniques in drug development, namely the choice of appropriate priors and computation of posterior probabilities. The computational issue has largely been solved thanks in part to the availability of efficient computational algorithms and high-speed computers. Notably, the introduction of the Markov chain Monte Carlo method (MCMC) (Gelfand and Smith 1990), and the development of the BUGS (Bayesian inference using Gibbs sampling) software (Lunn and Spiegelhalter 2009) were instrumental in promoting the routine application of the procedure. Nonetheless, since most Bayesian analyses tend to use computer-intensive algorithms or rely on extensive simulations to estimate trial- and model-operating characteristics, the implementation of the approaches may still be more cumbersome than the corresponding frequentist strategies. When appropriate, the computational burden may be minimized through use of conjugate priors or other techniques that are computationally less intensive (see, e.g., variational methods as used in Lee and Wand [2015]).

The second issue is the choice of appropriate priors. When the prior information is based mainly on subjective or personal opinion, the Bayesian approach may be controversial (FDA 2010). In drug development, it is now customary to inform the choice of the prior distribution based on data from previous trials or observational studies. A key assumption underlying the use of historical data to complement prior information is that of trial similarity or exchangeability. The assumption is not directly testable but requires careful assessment to ensure the appropriateness of the historical data to inform the construction of the prior distribution. This requires inputs from various stakeholders, including clinicians and statisticians, to ascertain that there are no substantial differences among the trials. It is especially important that if any deviation from exchangeability is suspected, use of suitable statistical models should be considered to perform appropriate correction (FDA 2010). For example, if the inter-trial difference is driven mainly by covariate imbalances, patient-level data, if available, may be used in the models to adjust for covariate imbalance (Pennello and Thompson 2008). In this setting, Bayesian hierarchical models are commonly used to provide estimates of parameters using data from heterogeneous sources (Braun and Wang 2010; Kwok and Lewis 2011).

Bayesian methods are useful to the sponsor earlier in the drug development process to arrive at go/no-go decisions. In this case a non-informative prior can be used to integrate with the likelihood. The posterior distribution can be used to make Bayesian probability statements on the parameter of interest to determine the go/no-go decision. This internal sponsor decision is not a regulatory concern.

In the following, we highlight a few relevant aspects of the application of Bayesian statistics in drug development, with special emphasis on the associated challenges in regulatory reviews.

2.6.2 Potential Areas of Application

In the recent past, Bayesian methods have been applied in the design and analyses of clinical trials in every stage of clinical development. The impact has especially been visible in areas where it is critical to enhance efficiency or when there are unmet medical needs.

In early development phases, Bayesian approaches are often used to implement adaptive dose-finding study designs, as opposed to the customary Phase I dose-escalation studies. One common approach in this regard, discussed elsewhere in this monograph, is the Continual Reassessment Method (CRM), which enables the estimation of the Maximum Tolerated Dose (MTD) using historical data, and data accumulated from previously studied doses (O'Quigley et al. 1990). Although the approach requires defining and implementing a suitable model to characterize the dose–response relationship, it is often preferred to rule-based methods, which may lack the rigor and reliability of CRMs.

Another potential application of Bayesian approaches is in the design of proof-of-concept studies, used in making important decisions about subsequent stages of a drug development program. Traditional Phase IIA trials often involve either a single arm, comparing a new drug against historical references, or a randomization scheme comparing the new drug with the standard treatment or placebo. Such fixed designs may not only unnecessarily expose patients to ineffective or toxic doses, but may also prolong the time to make go/no-go decisions. Bayesian adaptive designs may become viable options by allowing the use of accumulating data to inform decision to stop or continue a study in a stepwise fashion (Chung and Schultz 2007).

When there is interest to accelerate the drug development process, it is often proposed to integrate Phase II and Phase III programs seamlessly. This may be achieved using adaptive procedures to modify various aspects of the trial design, including doses, sample size, as well as development objectives (see, e.g., Schmidli et al. 2007). One feature of a seamless Phase II/III study design is that the final analyses will be based on data from both stages, typically in a Bayesian framework (Kimani et al. 2012). However, in the current regulatory framework it would be essential to ensure that the overall Type I error rate is controlled, and that there is strong evidence in support of the decision made at the end of the confirmatory stage.

As discussed in Section 2.5, adaptive designs are useful to enhance the efficiency of clinical trials, by incorporating flexibility in the design and conduct of the trial. One appealing feature of the Bayesian approach is the ability to incorporate accumulating or historical data to inform actions about various aspects of an ongoing trial while adhering to prespecified plans (FDA 2010). However, caution should be exercised in the implementation of these designs to mitigate the potential for operational bias. In particular, special effort should be made to ensure protection of type I error rates through extensive simulations (see, e.g., Spiegelhalter et al. 2000).

Evaluation of the safety of a drug based on postapproval data is often challenging due to the observational nature of the data, its high dimensionality, and the need to synthesize information from disparate sources. Bayesian approaches have been proposed as viable options for postapproval drug-safety signal detection, as they permit information borrowing from preapproval as well as across data sources and drug-adverse-effect combinations (Madigan et al. 2010). In addition, Type I error is not a concern in postapproval safety monitoring. However, Bayesian approaches are not solutions to other issues with such data, including confounding and other sources of bias.

In comparative effectiveness research, traditional and network meta-analysis methods are routinely used, since it is essential to combine studies from two or more trials to improve the precision of estimates of treatment effects or to perform indirect comparisons in cases where data from head-to-head RCTs is not available. Bayesian approaches have found appeal in such cases, since they permit the combining of information in a natural way (Greco et al. 2015).

2.6.3 Regulatory Considerations

Although the frequentist approach is predominantly used in trials intended for regulatory submissions, the role of Bayesian statistics in drug development is widely recognized by regulatory bodies (FDA 2010; ICH E9 Expert Working Group 1999). However, for a successful implementation of Bayesian methods in clinical trials, there should be upfront discussions and agreements between sponsors and the regulatory bodies about pertinent aspects of the approach, including the choice of priors, exchangeability of trials, and control of Type I error rates.

While the idea of controlling Type I error rates is central to the frequentist paradigm and is not an explicit feature of Bayesian decision-making, it is still of regulatory relevance, especially when informative priors are constructed using external information. Simulation experiments are generally required to assess Type I error rates, taking into consideration the pertinent features of the study design, including prior information, sample size, and any interim analyses planned or performed. It is generally recommended that the simulation involve alternative scenarios to provide adequate assurance about the estimated Type I error rate. In the event of inflated Type I error rate, it may be appropriate to take corrective measures, such as increasing the predictive probability of success, increasing the sample size to mitigate the influence of the prior, reducing the number of interim analyses, or discounting the prior information (see, e.g., FDA 2010).

The choice of priors is another cause for concern by regulatory agencies and advisory committees. Generally, subjective priors are difficult to justify. When historical data is used to inform priors, it is important to ensure that there is no selection bias in the choice of the data source. In some cases, the historical data may have been selected omitting unfavorable data for the study drug. This may be due to logistical constraints, especially when there are legal constraints to obtain prior information or possibly a publication bias, if data are taken from the literature. When the information from historical data appears to be dominant, it may be worthwhile to discount the prior through suitable criteria. Some approaches for discounting priors include increasing the sample size of the new trial, reducing the number of patients "borrowed" from the historical control, weighting the historical data, and employing hierarchical models with conservative hyper parameters (FDA 2010). An alternative strategy, is the use of the power prior, which incorporates a parameter κ ($0 \leq \kappa \leq 1$) that is intended to adjust the influence of the external information, especially in situations where there is imbalance in sample sizes or heterogeneity among studies (Zellner 1988). Technically, the power prior distribution is a product of the prior before the historical data was collected and the likelihood function of the historical data, the latter raised to the power *of* κ. Since the choice of κ requires a thorough understanding of the influence of the external information, it is good practice to perform extensive sensitivity analyses in order to understand the impact of different values of κ, ranging from 0 (non-informative) to 1 (full borrowing). Detailed discussions of various aspects of power priors may be found, among others, in Ibrahim et al. (2015).

The assumption of exchangeability or consistency between the current study and historical studies is not directly testable, and it may not be straightforward to validate. This is especially concerning when using hierarchical models in which prior information is obtained from only one historical study, since it is not possible to get an estimate of inter-study variability. As reported earlier, if the various sources of data are not exchangeable, the consequence might be reduced power, inflation of Type I error rate, or biased estimates (Viele et al. 2014). Typically, exchangeability should be assessed at the planning stage based on various statistical, clinical, and manufacturing considerations. For example, one statistical approach involves computing the posterior predictive probability of observing a discrepancy in the value of a given outcome between the current study and historical studies at least as large as that observed, under exchangeability (Pennello and Thompson 2008).

2.6.4 Challenges with Bayesian Statistics

One of the major impediments for wider use of Bayesian methods in drug development is the lack of a clear regulatory framework for its acceptance in the drug-approval process. While there are positive steps in that direction, such as the FDA guideline for use of Bayesian statistics in devices (FDA 2010), most of the widely referenced guidelines, including ICH E9 (ICH E9 Expert Working Group 1999), give greater emphasis to frequentist approaches.

Bayesian trials also have certain inherent difficulties that may make them less appealing to clinical trialists. For example, it may require substantial effort to prespecify some important decisions at the design stage, including the choice of the prior information, and how it would be incorporated with the trial data. Further, despite the considerable progress made in the implementation of Bayesian models, the approach is still computationally intensive compared to corresponding frequentist techniques, especially the requirement to perform extensive simulations to assess the operating characteristics of the procedure. Nevertheless, Bayesian reasoning parallels human thinking, i.e., what we know about the parameter of interest going into an experiment and how the experimental results change our knowledge.

2.6.5 Concluding Remarks

Despite the growing interest in Bayesian statistics, the broader application of the approach has not been fully realized. In this section, we highlighted some of the opportunities and challenges from regulatory and drug-development perspectives. With the increasing focus on enhancing the efficiency of clinical trials, Bayesian methods will arguably continue to garner acceptability, especially given their role in facilitating decision-making through use of historical and accumulating data.

2.7 SURROGATE ENDPOINTS AND BIOMARKERS

2.7.1 Introduction

The FDA-NIH Biomarker Working Group (2016) defines a biomarker as a "characteristic that is measured as an indicator of normal biological processes, pathogenic processes, or responses to an exposure or intervention, including therapeutic interventions." It is noted that there is a clear distinction between biomarkers and clinical outcome assessments (COAs), which typically relate to how an individual feels or functions, or how long the person lives. COAs are measured using a report generated by a clinician, patient, non-clinician observer, or a performance-based assessment, and, unlike biomarkers, can be used to quantify treatment effect in a clinical trial. Different types of biomarkers may be defined, depending on their intended use. For example, the so-called predictive biomarkers help to identify patients that are likely to benefit from or be harmed by a treatment option. On the other hand, prognostic biomarkers help to assess the likelihood of a clinical event, including disease recurrence or progression. In certain situations, pharmacodynamic biomarkers may be used to determine the occurrence of a biological response to treatment in an individual. Other categories include predisposition or susceptibility biomarkers, used in the determination of the risk of developing a disease; and diagnostic biomarkers, concerned with the identification of individuals with the disease or condition of interest. The development of biomarkers involves adherence to strict regulatory requirements. This entails obtaining qualification that is based on robust evidence that demonstrates the biomarkers are fit for purpose in drug development and evaluation. Once a biomarker is qualified, it has the potential to provide critical information to enhance clinical-trial design and facilitate the regulatory review process.

In personalized medicine, certain molecular targeted therapies tend to involve a high cost of delivery. In such instances, use of biomarkers that predict response may be a viable alternative to gain efficiency. This is especially attractive, provided the cost associated with the use of companion diagnostics, which involves testing before giving treatment, is not in excess of the savings obtained by tailoring treatment only to the target patient population.

Surrogate endpoints relate to a small class of biomarkers that serve as a substitute for clinical outcomes, which directly measure how patients feel, function, or survive. Surrogate endpoints are particularly preferred when the desired clinical outcomes are not readily obtainable for practical or ethical reasons. Thus, the primary function of a surrogate endpoint is to predict, but not measure, clinical benefit or harm. However, the validity and reliability of a surrogate endpoint must first be established before it can be used in medical research or clinical practice. This requires extensive testing to see how well they predict, or correlate with, clinical benefit. In general, the predictive capacity of a surrogate endpoint is evaluated based on data from a variety of sources, including epidemiologic, therapeutic, pathophysiologic, or other scientific experiments. Depending on the level of clinical validation, surrogate endpoints may be classified as candidate, reasonably likely, or validated. Surrogate endpoints are considered candidate when they are still under evaluation for their predictive ability, whereas reasonably likely surrogate endpoints require support based on strong mechanistic and/or epidemiologic rationale.

In general, there is no definitive way of establishing the validity of a given biomarker as a surrogate endpoint. However, there are a few surrogate endpoints that are now in routine use, both in the context of drug approval and medical practice. Examples include HbA1c, a measure of glycemic control, which is a surrogate for disease severity and outcomes of morbidity and mortality in patients with diabetes; and serum cholesterol levels (e.g., LDL-C), which serves as a surrogate for similar cardiovascular outcomes.

In the following sections, we highlight statistical and regulatory issues that are of relevance to the use of biomarkers and surrogate endpoints in drug development. Special emphasis is given to the requirements for validating and qualification of biomarkers and surrogate endpoints, and the resources available to facilitate the development of biomarkers by sponsors.

2.7.2 Statistical Considerations

From a statistical perspective, the analysis of biomarkers and surrogate endpoints is associated with several challenges, including the assessment of the validity and clinical utility of the marker, as well as the handling of high dimensionality and multiplicity issues. Recent advances in modern analytic methods and new-generation sequencing appear to address some of the issues, but this is an active area of research with considerable opportunities to advance drug development and evidence-based medicine (Matsui 2013).

When dealing with one biomarker at a time, traditional univariate techniques can serve as screening tools. Advantages of such approaches include ease of implementation of the procedures and interpretation of the results. A major drawback is the inability to utilize the potential correlations among biomarkers. Therefore, it may often be essential to use more sophisticated multivariate methods when dealing with several biomarkers. Most traditional approaches may not be suitable to handle multivariate biomarker data, especially when dealing with such issues as the high dimensions, missing values, multicollinearity, and multiplicity. Accordingly, modern analytical approaches, including penalized regression, decision trees, and neural networks, may need to be considered (see, e.g., Hastie et al. 2009). In genomics, for example, hierarchical models can be used, since such models draw strength by incorporating information across comparable genes (see, e.g., Speed 2003).

After a promising set of genes or markers is identified, one may then assess the diagnostic potential of the markers using alternative models, while incorporating additional clinical information. Lu et al. (2013) report results that are based on the use of a penalized-regression approach to analyze data from an AIDS trial. In DeRubeis et al. (2014), a linear regression model has been applied to develop an individual treatment rule utilizing data from an RCT.

In association analyses involving many markers, one needs to control the possibility of false positives. Traditional approaches, such as the Bonferroni method tend to be too strict and may lead to many missed findings. The false discovery rate (FDR), defined as the expected proportion of incorrectly rejected null hypotheses among the declared significant results, was introduced by Benjamini and Hochberg (1995) as an attractive alternative to the more conservative traditional methods for simultaneous inference. Subsequent enhancements of the FDR include the positive false discovery rate (pFDR) and the q-value, which is a measure of significance in terms of the FDR rather than the usual false positive rate associated with traditional p-values (Storey and Tibshirani 2003).

As pointed out earlier, before a biomarker can be used in practice, its validity and reliability have to rigorously be assessed and established. A common approach, often referred to as analytical validation, is to use a gold standard to determine the reliability of the assay and the sensitivity and specificity of the measurements (Chau et al. 2008). In contrast, clinical validity relates to the assessment of the predictive value of a biomarker for disease prognosis or treatment effect. When the focus is on prognostic biomarkers, clinical validation requires the determination of the strength of correlation between biomarker values and a clinical endpoint.

In the context of randomized controlled trials (RCTs), clinical validity of a predictive biomarker may be evaluated with respect to the degree of significance of the treatment-by-biomarker interaction in a suitable model. Further, it is important to establish the clinical utility of the biomarker, i.e., whether the use of the biomarker in clinical practice has benefits. This is often accomplished through suitably designed clinical trials. One approach involves randomizing patients either to a standard of care therapy or to a strategy in which a biomarker-based treatment assignment is used. In other cases, enrichment designs may be employed in which treatment effect is assessed using only patients who are predicted to be responders based on the biomarker under consideration (Matsui 2013; Simon 2010).

When the intent is to determine whether biomarkers can serve as a surrogate for a clinical endpoint, it is essential to evaluate a number of conditions with the help of suitable statistical techniques. The exercise typically involves an assessment of the effect of the drug on the biomarker, the effect of the drug on the clinical endpoint of interest, and the association of the surrogate biomarker and the clinical endpoint. In a seminal work, Prentice (1989) introduced an approach under the assumption that "a response variable for which a test of the null hypothesis of no relationship to the treatment groups under comparison is also a valid test of the corresponding null hypothesis based on the true endpoint." Implicit in the criterion is that the surrogate response variable captures all the information pertaining to the relationship between the treatment and the true endpoint. In other words, given the surrogate endpoint, the impact of treatment is conditionally independent of the true endpoint. One of the drawbacks of Prentice's approach is its reliance on untestable assumptions. Clearly, conditioning on the surrogate, which is obtained posttreatment, is noncausal. Further, as argued in Berger (2004), the criterion provides a necessary, but not sufficient, condition to infer a treatment effect on the true endpoint.

Since Prentice's idea of perfect surrogacy is unrealistic, Freedman et al. (1992) and Wang and Taylor (2003) introduced an approach based on the proportion of treatment effect explained. However, the approach still relies on conditioning on a posttreatment marker, and it may also lead to ratio estimates that may lie outside the acceptable limits of 0 to 1 and having high variability.

An alternative strategy involves combining information from several trials, with a view to assessing the "trial level association" between the treatment effect on the surrogate and the treatment effect on the true endpoint (Buyse et al. 2015). An example of the application of the meta-analytic approach may be found in Paoletti et al. (2013), in which results are reported concerning the validity of progression-free survival as a surrogate for overall survival in advanced/recurrent gastric cancer trials.

Although the meta-analytic approach appears attractive, in practice it may not be feasible to get data from multiple sources on a biomarker and a new treatment. Therefore, ongoing research is still needed for establishing the reliability of surrogate markers intended for use in drug development and clinical practice.

2.7.3 Regulatory Considerations

The importance of qualified biomarkers to provide valuable information that can help reduce uncertainty in regulatory decisions is well-recognized. Accordingly, regulatory agencies have established strict guidelines for the qualification process of biomarkers. In the US, the *21st Century Cures Act* describes the process to develop a biomarker for regulatory use. To help sponsors with the development of biomarkers, the US FDA also has several resources, including the Biomarker Qualification Program, through which developers may request regulatory qualification of a biomarker for use in drug development (FDA 2018a).

When a new biomarker is proposed for use as a surrogate endpoint, the US FDA uses the type C meeting process to engage sponsors in discussions around the feasibility and limitations of the surrogate as a primary efficacy endpoint. Incidentally, the FDA is required by law to make public a list of "surrogate endpoints which were the basis of approval or licensure (as applicable) of a drug or biological product" (FDA 2018a). The information, which is updated periodically, is expected to facilitate discussions between sponsors and the FDA on the use of potential surrogate endpoints. It should be underscored that a surrogate endpoint that is validated for a specific pharmacologic class of treatment regimens is not necessarily valid as a surrogate endpoint for other classes of drugs. Indeed, the acceptability of a surrogate marker is context-dependent, relying on several factors, including the disease, patient population, therapeutic mechanism of action, and availability of current treatments (FDA 2018a).

The US FDA relies on the accelerated-approval regulatory process to enhance the accessibility of medicines to patients with unmet needs, especially for conditions leading to death or serious illness. The process involves granting approvals to market interventions that demonstrate strong effects with respect to reasonably likely surrogate endpoints, i.e., reasonably likely to predict a clinical benefit. This implies that the evidentiary strength of the effect of treatment on the surrogate must be strong. The approval is granted with a requirement that the sponsors also conduct postapproval clinical trials to show that these markers can be relied upon to predict, or correlate with, clinical benefit. However, as argued in Fleming (2005), the use of such surrogate markers in accelerated approvals requires addressing important operational challenges, including timely completion of the postapproval commitment trials, to protect the best interest of public health.

The European Medicines Agency (EMA) also provides several guidelines relating to the qualification of biomarkers, highlighting important points to consider that have been identified as common and major challenges and limitations (EMA 2017a). A successful qualification process presupposes adequate demonstration of diagnostic and prognostic performance, predictive value for clinical outcome, as well as sensitivity to detect change reflecting the clinical status of patients. In addition, the guidelines stress that the study design and statistical methodology to be used must be prespecified, and that the clinical utility and the appropriateness of the analytical platform should be justified.

2.7.4 Concluding Remarks

The development of reliable and valid biomarkers is a critical component of drug development and regulatory review. In this section, we highlighted several statistical and regulatory issues associated with the development and qualification of biomarkers. When used as a surrogate endpoint, a biomarker serves as a substitute for a clinical endpoint, which directly quantifies clinical benefit or harm. Therefore, the development of a biomarker as a surrogate endpoint should also undergo a process consisting of analytical validation based on extensive documentation, and subsequent qualification by a regulatory body.

While the main emphasis in this section is on biomarkers that can be used as surrogate endpoints, there is also a growing interest in the use of biomarkers to enrich clinical trials, with a view to enhancing the efficiency of drug development and advancing the field of precision medicine. Such strategies may restrict inclusion of patients with a specified biomarker (to reduce variability), patients in high risk categories (prognostic enrichment), or patients who are more likely to respond to the study drug (predictive enrichment) (FDA 2019).

Finally, under certain circumstances, especially in the absence of evidence on relevant clinical endpoint that directly measures clinical benefit, surrogate endpoints can be acceptable for relative effectiveness assessment (REA) in pricing and reimbursement negotiations. As outlined in a recently issued guideline, acceptability of surrogate endpoints for REA requires equally rigorous scientific and clinical knowledge for the qualification of biomarkers as surrogate endpoints (EUnetHTA 2013). This includes demonstration of the relationships between the surrogate and the clinical endpoint based on biological plausibility and empirical evidence. In addition, the guideline recommends that the level of evidence, the associated uncertainties, and any limitations of their use should be explicitly explained. Further, it is noted that if a surrogate endpoint has already been adequately validated, it is not essential to carry out additional validation just for REA purposes.

2.8 SUBGROUP ANALYSES

2.8.1 Introduction

The analysis of subgroups in confirmatory clinical trials encompasses many statistical and regulatory issues. These issues include multiplicity, inflation of Type 1 error, estimation and interpretation of treatment effects in subgroups, *ad hoc* nature of some subgroup findings, and the regulatory requirement to assess the consistency of the treatment effect within the study population. These issues are clearly interrelated and sometimes at odds with each other from both statistical and regulatory perspectives. The issue of subgroup analyses also touches on the important area of innovative clinical-trial designs; for example, within oncology, analyses informed by biomarkers or targeted therapy based on a specific genetic mutation among a larger class of tumors. The growing trend toward personalized medicine and targeted therapies, as well as the prescription and payment of treatments by physicians and insurers, respectively, all make subgroup design and interpretation one of the more important current areas of statistical and regulatory interaction. European Medicines Agency (2019) has issued guidance specific to subgroup analysis in clinical trials. While FDA has not issued a general subgroup guidance, it has issued one specific to clinical trials for medical devices pertaining to age, race and ethnicity (see FDA 2017a). FDA has also released a guidance on medical communications that are consistent with the FDA-required labeling that recognizes the importance of communication of subgroup results (FDA 2018b). The various issues around subgroup analyses will be discussed from the traditional perspective and from the changing regulatory landscape.

2.8.2 Subgroup Analyses in the Traditional Confirmatory Clinical-Trial Setting

The traditional clinical trial is designed to show a treatment benefit in a target population. This target population is comprised of clinically important subgroups; for example, sex, race, age, baseline disease severity, etc. There is a regulatory imperative to assess the consistency of the treatment effect across important subgroups. This can be addressed by an analysis of the interaction effect for subgroup by treatment or analyses of the treatment effect within subgroups or both. While there is a need to address consistency, the definition of consistency and the interpretation of results are ambiguous. The regulatory purpose of these analyses is to provide support to the conclusion of an overall significant treatment effect in the population of interest and to assess whether there are any subpopulations in which the treatment may not be effective, for example, a qualitative interaction of treatment with baseline severity.

A confirmatory clinical trial is powered to detect a treatment effect in the overall target population. It is not powered to detect interactions or to detect treatment effects within subgroups, unless the subgroup is intended to be part of the approved label as discussed in the next section. These subgroup analyses conducted under the regulatory imperative are descriptive rather than inferential from a statistical perspective, even though regulators may draw inferences in the review process. Thus, the issue of multiplicity and the need to specify a multiple-testing procedure are not typically applicable at the design stage for this category of subgroup analyses. However, the estimation and interpretation of treatment effects in subgroups are important to the proper interpretation of the clinical trial results. The prespecification of specific subgroups in the protocol should be limited to those where there is some *apriori* evidence of clinical importance. By default, any *ad hoc* findings in subgroups outside of the prespecified set are only exploratory findings and have to be interpreted with a great deal of caution. Estimates of subgroup treatment effects should not be interpreted on their face values. Even with the subgroup being prespecified, there remains the question of whether the subgroup-specific estimate or the overall population estimate is the better estimate of treatment effect within the subgroup. It is well-known that estimates can vary considerably over subgroups given the same underlying treatment effect. To address the potential of overinterpretation of subgroup differences, the magnitude of the difference, the biological and mechanistic plausibility of the difference, and the clinical importance of the difference should be considered. In addition, estimation methods, such as empirical Bayes that takes into account the overall-population treatment effect in the estimation of the subgroup effect, should be considered.

2.8.3 Statistical Approaches

Traditional subgroup analysis typically involves the use of linear or generalized linear models to test the interaction between treatment and a subgroup as well as the significance of the treatment effect within the subgroups (Pocock et al. 2002). When the treatment-by-subgroup interaction is significant, it is customary to assess the nature of the interaction, i.e., whether it is qualitative or quantitative (Gail and Simon 1985). In the case of the former, in which the treatment effect varies both in magnitude and direction in the various subgroups, a general statement cannot be made about the overall result. However, caution should still be exercised in presenting an estimate of an overall treatment effect even when the interaction is of a quantitative nature, since the degree of benefit or harm may not be similar across subgroups.

The reliability of results based on linear or generalized linear models is heavily dependent on the plausibility of the underlying assumptions, including the functional form, absence of multicollinearity, and parsimony of the model relative to the available sample size. To mitigate some of the associated issues, alternative techniques have been proposed, including classification and regression trees (CART) and penalized regression.

CART and other recursive-partitioning approaches are typically used for exploratory analyses and are appealing in that they do not require specification of the usual linear-model assumptions (Breiman et al. 1984; Su et al. 2009). More recently, subgroup identification methods have been proposed that are based on differential-effect searches (see, e.g., Foster et al. 2011). In the presence of multicollinearity and model sparsity, alternative penalized-regression approaches have been proposed, including least absolute shrinkage and selection operator (LASSO) and other related techniques (Hastie et al. 2009).

As reported in a recent study (Alemayehu et al. 2018), the performance of the techniques is dependent on a number of factors, including sample size, correlation among covariates, subgroup sizes, and interaction magnitudes. For most practical applications, especially those involving regulatory submissions, the traditional approaches are adequate. However, looking forward on the regulatory landscape, in situations where the dimension of the predictors is large relative to the sample size, modern techniques, particularly machine learning and other data-mining methods, may be required. For exploratory analyses, where prespecification is not practical, data-driven strategies may be utilized to select the most appropriate technique for a given situation.

2.8.4 Reporting and Interpretation of Subgroup Results

In view of the inherent issues with subgroup analyses, including multiplicity and power, results should be interpreted with caution, and reported with full transparency and fair balance (Wang et al. 2007). When the results are based on prespecified analyses, all favorable and unfavorable findings should be provided, accompanied by details of the statistical approaches employed, including multiplicity adjustment, magnitude of treatment effects, and sample size.

When interesting results are observed from *ad hoc* analyses, it is critical to disclose the total number of analyses performed, the comparability of treatment groups within subgroups with respect to relevant prognostic factors, and the consistency of the findings with other similar trials or the known mechanism of action or biology of the drug or therapeutic area.

2.8.5 Subgroup Analyses in the Changing Clinical-Trial and Regulatory Setting

The importance of subgroup analyses has increased due to heightened interests by regulators, healthcare providers and payers, patients and patient advocacy groups, and researchers and medical journals. This heightened interest is motivated by basic biological research that has led to the recognition that the true treatment effect may be quite different among subgroups even to the extent of working in only one subgroup. Consequently, the relatively new concepts of targeted therapies and personalized medicine have emerged in drug development. This is particularly prominent in cancer therapy in which specific biomarkers or genetic mutations are used for targeted therapies. The importance of identifying, say in a breast cancer study, a patient who responds to treatment, or conversely who does not, is obvious. Regulators need to properly label the treatment; prescribers and payers want to know the type of patient with an expected benefit from the treatment; and, certainly, the individual patient wants to know whether the treatment has been shown to be effective in their tumor. Thus, subgroup analyses are essential to interpret the results of clinical trials in which the treatment may or may not be effective in the overall disease population. However, to establish efficacy within a subgroup with a particular biomarker or genetic mutation out of a more general tumor-type in the same clinical trial, or to establish efficacy in more than one cancer site requires prespecification of hypotheses in the protocol along with a multiple-testing procedure to control Type 1 error (see Section 2.1 for more discussion on multiplicity).

These issues can be addressed more efficiently in innovative clinical-trial designs, such as basket trials or platform trials. For example, there may be multiple cancers with the same molecular target, where within each basket (subgroup) a different tumor site is studied within the same trial. It is evident that there are multiple pathways across subgroups to a positive trial and that the use of such a design for a confirmatory trial requires a clear analysis plan and control of Type 1 error (see Section 2.5.2 for more discussion on basket trials).

The importance of subgroup findings is also motivated by the desire of patients, prescribers, and payers to have adequate knowledge of the efficacy and safety of a drug in patients with specific characteristics. For example, one may be interested in understanding how the treatment performs in an elderly population or with severe disease. In multiregional studies, FDA or EMA would be interested in how the treatment performs in subgroups of patients within the scope of their regulatory authority. Clinical trials are not generally designed with sufficient power to address these questions definitively, nevertheless, the results may be informative. FDA has released a guidance, "Medical product communications that are consistent with the FDA-required labeling" (FDA 2018b), which recognizes that sponsors want to promote data about approved uses of their products that are not contained in the product labeling and that this promotion is useful. An area specifically addressed in the document is patient subgroups. This guidance indicates greater acceptance by FDA of subgroup findings that do not generally rise to the level of the new drug-approval standard of "substantial evidence." However, any presentation of subgroup results will be scrutinized under the "misleading impression" criterion. Furthermore, the findings or conclusions cannot be overstated or fail to disclose their material limitations. Without the requirement of substantial evidence, the contextual language is very important in order that subgroup results be viewed as descriptive rather than inferential.

2.8.6 Conclusion

The efficacy and safety of a treatment in subgroups of the population for which the drug is approved is important. There is a regulatory requirement to assess the consistency of a treatment's performance within important subgroups. There is a growing recognition that the knowledge of subgroup findings is desired by patients, prescribers, payers, sponsors, and regulators. The statistical issues with subgroup analyses are well-known and include multiplicity and effect-size estimation. With multiple subgroup analyses, the play of chance is large, and the interpretation of subgroup effects must keep chance in mind so as not to overinterpret subgroup findings. The magnitude of the difference in the subgroup, the biological and mechanistic plausibility of the difference, and the clinical importance of the difference should also be considered. In general, subgroup results should be viewed as descriptive and not inferential. Of course, there may be the goal of establishing efficacy in a targeted subgroup among a larger population in a confirmatory clinical trial, as may be the case in some innovative designs. In this case the prespecification of hypotheses in the protocol along with a multiple-testing procedure to control the overall Type 1 error is required for inferential purposes.

2.9 BENEFIT–RISK ASSESSMENT

2.9.1 Introduction

Following the approval of a new drug by regulatory authorities, the evaluation of the benefits and risks continues throughout the lifecycle of the product. This typically consists of a transparent synthesis and communication of data from diverse sources relating to the drug's effectiveness, safety, tolerability, and patient preference. Since the effort involves extracting and integrating information from a large amount of heterogenous data, regulatory agencies have established guidelines and other appropriate mechanisms to ensure appropriate analysis, interpretation, and communication of the benefit–risk profiles of authorized drugs, with a view to protecting public health and advancing health outcomes (Guo et al. 2010).

There have also been parallel initiatives undertaken by the pharmaceutical industry to align with the expectations of the regulators with respect to the enhancement of the approaches for assessment of the benefit–risk of medicines. In the US, the Pharmaceutical Research and Manufacturers of America (PhRMA) initially developed the so-called Benefit–Risk Action Team (BRAT) Framework, which was eventually transferred to the Centre for Innovation in Regulatory Science (CIRS), a neutral independent UK-based subsidiary company (Levitan 2012). Efforts have also been underway to establish good-practice guidelines for conducting agencies to aid healthcare decision-making (Thokala et al. 2016).

Despite the numerous efforts and initiatives by both regulators and pharmaceutical companies, there is still a demand for a standard template to harmonize the evaluation of the benefit–risk profiles of drugs and the documentation and communication of decisions. The Universal Methodologies for Benefit–Risk Assessment (UMBRA) is an example of a framework proposed by representatives of regulators and the pharmaceutical industry, with the aim of establishing common elements of an overarching, internationally acceptable, standardized benefit–risk approach (Centre for Innovation in Regulatory Science 2012).

In this section, we highlight pertinent methodological and regulatory issues relating to the benefit–risk assessment of medicinal products and provide a summary of selected tools that are currently accepted for use by sponsors and regulatory agencies.

2.9.2 Methodological Considerations in Benefit–Risk Analysis

Broadly, benefit–risk assessment may be carried out either in a descriptive/qualitative or quantitative framework. Descriptive approaches typically use metrics for structuring relevant benefits and risks and involve a thorough assessment of treatment performance data on benefits, risks, and convenience of use, without applying weights. On the other hand, quantitative approaches aim at combining data on treatment effectiveness, safety, and ease of use, with stakeholder preference information, typically using a weighting scheme for various benefit and risk criteria. Preference-based approaches are generally applicable in complex situations involving several criteria and multiple treatment options. Some of the widely used quantitative approaches permit integration of data into a single measure, thereby facilitating and ensuring transparent communication of benefit–risk decisions. However, these quantitative methods may obscure the underlying data and may not be necessary if the more direct qualitative and graphical summaries are clear.

Development of a quantitative model requires determination of appropriate benefit and risk criteria, which relate to distinct and nonoverlapping clinical outcomes of interest for the treatment options under consideration. Estimates of drug performance on each criterion should then be obtained, including the associated measures of uncertainties of the estimators. When data comes just from a single RCT, the performance measures may be computed and analyzed with either a frequentist or Bayesian approach. In certain cases, data may be available from multiple trials, in which case the relevant information may be combined using methods for standard meta-analysis or network meta-analysis, depending on whether a common comparator is available or not.

A major issue associated with the analysis of data to establish the benefit–risk profile of a drug is the quantification of the uncertainty and the clinical relevance of the observed effect sizes. This in part is because the data used in benefit–risk assessment may come from diverse sources, including RCTs, epidemiology studies, literature review, or spontaneous adverse reports. Further, the uncertainty may arise in at least two other ways, namely, in the subjective choice of the criteria, or as a consequence of sampling variability. In the latter case, the handling of sampling variability requires application of suitable statistical methods. On the other hand, subjective uncertainty generally requires execution of extensive sensitivity analyses.

A commonly used quantitative approach for benefit–risk assessment is the multiple-criteria decision analysis (MCDA) method, introduced by Keeney and Raiffa (1976). It involves a decision-making process that brings together different options on multiple criteria of benefits and risks into an overall assessment, through scoring and weighting. The purpose of scoring is to quantify each criterion into a common scale, while weighting ensures comparability of the units on the criteria so that they can be combined into an overall scale. More specifically, suppose the mean of the ith criterion is denoted by μ_i, with an associated score function and weight, s_i and w_i, respectively. Then a measure of an overall assessment is given by:

$$\vartheta = \sum w_i s_i \left(\mu_i\right)$$

Inference about ϑ can be made by replacing μ_i with a suitable estimator. Approximate confidence intervals and test statistics may be constructed using the central limit theorem or via simulations.

An attractive feature of the MCDA approach is that it permits combining the subjective value judgments and the clinical evidence in a transparent fashion. However, its limitations include the fact that it does not handle uncertainties of outcomes and, most importantly, that it requires exact specification of the values of the preferences and weights.

To mitigate the limitations of the standard MCDA method, enhanced approaches have been proposed, assuming distributions, rather than point values, for the weights and score functions. One example is the approach proposed by Tervonen et al. (2011), dubbed the stochastic multicriteria acceptability analysis (SMAA), which is intended to account for the uncertainty in the criterion measurements as well as preferences information. More specifically, the approach assumes the weights and the criteria are random variables with joint density functions. A rank acceptability index is then computed as a multidimensional integral over the criteria distributions and the favorable rank weights.

In the above SMAA framework, estimation of the distribution of the criteria is often challenging. Waddingham et al. (2016) proposed an approach that involves a synthesis of the evidence from other studies. Saint-Hilary et al. (2017) provided a method for constructing the weight space of SMAA. More recently, Li et al. (2018) introduced a framework in which Bayesian meta-analysis and SMAA are jointly used to synthesize accumulating evidence from early stages of the clinical development to late stages in benefit–risk assessment.

Software programs are available for implementation of some of the abovementioned techniques. In R, the CRAN packages, *hitandrun* and SMAA can be used to implement the methods. In addition, the Aggregate Data Drug Information System (ADDIS) software can be used for both SMAA and MCDA (van Valkenhoef et al. 2013).

In addition to the structured qualitative and quantitative approaches mentioned above, there are several semi-quantitative techniques that are in routine use, depending on the scenario at hand. Examples include such procedures as number needed to treat (NNT), number needed to harm (NNH), decision trees, and Markov models. While NNT and NNH are measures that are apparently easy to interpret, they are based on the inverse of the risk difference with often wide upper-confidence bounds and thus should not be presented without the confidence limits. A detailed description of the approaches may be found, e.g., in EMA (2010a).

Lastly, as pointed out earlier, sensitivity analyses are an essential component of benefit–risk assessment to establish the robustness of the results against the treatment performance or preference estimates. This may involve either evaluating one parameter at a time or several parameters simultaneously. The latter often entails defining suitable distributions to the parameters, as is the case in the SMAA approach described above.

2.9.3 Regulatory Perspectives

One of the most important aspects of regulatory decision-making is the assessment and communication of the risks and benefits of medicinal products in a transparent and structured manner. This is highlighted in the recent guidance formulated by the International Council for Harmonization of Technical Requirements for Pharmaceuticals for Human Use (ICH), as part of the revisions to its guidance document M4E: The CTD – Efficacy (ICH 2016). The updated document provides flexibility and general recommendations for formatting and structuring benefit–risk assessments, without any explicit suggestion for or against specific methodologies or approaches.

In 2005 the US FDA issued a framework for the pharmaceutical industry that consisted of guidelines for premarketing risk assessment, development, and use of risk minimization action plans, and good pharmacovigilance practices and pharmacoepidemiologic assessment (Guo et al. 2010). Subsequently, the agency developed an enhanced framework for benefit–risk assessment to provide a "structured, qualitative approach focused on identifying and clearly communicating key issues, evidence, and uncertainties in FDA's benefit–risk assessment and how those considerations inform regulatory decisions" (FDA 2013). As depicted in Figure 2.5, the Benefit–Risk Framework (BRF) outlines the critical elements that are relevant for the benefit–risk assessment and provides specifications for describing the evidence and uncertainties as well as the conclusions and reasons for each dimension. Further, it gives an integrated summary of the assessment, with a succinct explanation and rationale for regulatory decisions.

On behalf of the European Medicines Agency (EMA), the Committee for Medicinal Products for Human Use (CHMP) has also issued similar guidelines, including an assessment of the potential value of existing benefit–risk models and methods (Guo et al. 2010). In 2010, the EMA sponsored the Benefit–Risk Methodology Project, which reviewed several qualitative and quantitative approaches, and proposed PROACT-URL

Benefit-Risk Integrated Assessment		
Benefit-Risk Dimensions		
Dimension	Evidence and Uncertainties	Conclusions and Reasons
Analysis of Condition		
Current Treatment Options		
Benefit		
Risk and Risk Management		

FIGURE 2.5 FDA Benefit–Risk Framework

Source: www.fda.gov/media/112570/download (Accessed on June 9, 2019)

(Problem formulation, Objectives, Alternatives Consequences, Tradeoffs, Uncertainties, Risk tolerance, Linked decisions) (EMA 2010a). The agency's emphasis on benefit–risk assessment was further reinforced in the so-called Roadmap-to-2015 framework, in which the benefit–risk balance assessment model was identified as one of the strategic areas (EMA 2011). A related unit that the EMA coordinates is the European Network of Centers for Pharmacoepidemiology and Pharmacovigilance (ENCePP), which primarily focuses on the strengthening of the evaluation of the benefit–risk balance of medicines through the conduct of high-quality observational studies.

The EMA introduced the so-called Effects Table with a view to enhancing the consistency, transparency, and communication of benefit–risk assessments (EMA 2015). The table, displayed in Figure 2.6, presents effects and information for the benefit–risk balance, and allows incorporation of results based on quantitative methods.

Efforts are also under way in other countries, such as Australia, to develop a framework for effective assessment and communication of benefits vs. risks of medicines.

Recently, regulatory bodies have shown keen interest in incorporating patient preferences in making decisions. In the US, there are several FDA

Effect	Short Description	Unit	Treatment	Control	Uncertainties/ Strength of evidence	References
Favourable						
Unfavourable						

FIGURE 2.6 EMA Effects Table

Source: EMA. Guidance document on the content of the Rapporteur day 80 critical-assessment report. Overview and lists of question. 2015. EMA/90842/2015. Available from www.ema.europa.eu/docs/en_GB/document_library/Regulatory_and_procedural_guideline/2009/10/WC500004800.pdf.

guidance documents that provide specific suggestions on integrating patient preferences into benefit–risk assessments. Further, the *21st Century Cures Act* and the Prescription Drug User Fee Act, Revision VI (PDUFA VI) of the FDA Reauthorization Act highlight the importance of considering the patient experience during the drug-development process. In Europe, similar initiatives are under way, including a collaborative project known as The Pharmacoepidemiological Research on Outcomes of Therapeutics by a European Consortium (PROTECT), which is concerned with the exploration of how preferences can be incorporated into the decision-making process (Hughes et al. 2016).

2.9.4 Benefit–Risk in Health-Technology Assessment

Some of the approaches, including the MCDA, have also been applied in health-technology assessment (HTA) decisions. HTA is a framework employed in several countries for the purpose of making reimbursement decisions for new technologies, applying agreed-upon principles and criteria. HTA bodies in several countries, such as Germany, England, Australia, and Thailand, leverage MCDA approaches in coverage decision-making (Thokala et al. 2016). Although the approaches tend to differ among the various HTA systems, there are certain elements that are common to many of them, including the incorporation of data on effectiveness, patient need, and burden of disease.

One area that seems to be a point of contention is the consideration of cost and budget impact as factors in the implementation of MCDA models in HTA. In addition, the quantitative incorporation of patient preference data in HTAs is not as well-established as it is in benefit–risk assessment (Mott 2018). This is often attributed to the limitations of the commonly used methods in HTA, such as cost-utility analysis, which only focus on eliciting health-state utilities from patients. In this respect, MCDAs may provide an attractive alternative (Angelis 2017).

2.9.5 Concluding Remarks

In this section, we provided a high-level overview of benefit–risk assessment methods and the associated issues. A balanced assessment of the benefits and risks of a drug presupposes a synthesis of stakeholder preference with quality evidence on effectiveness and safety and communicating the results in a transparent and succinct manner. Accordingly, there have been important achievements in recent years by regulators that include frameworks to enhance the process of benefit–risk decision-making. In addition, pharmaceutical companies routinely institute risk evaluation and mitigation strategies for their prescription drugs, and coordinate efforts with regulatory bodies to align approaches.

Notwithstanding the availability of guidelines and reporting tools, there is still a need to develop a harmonized framework to enhance the assessment and communication of benefits and risks. Although, qualitative approaches appear to be preferred by some regulatory bodies and other stakeholders, the role of quantitative approaches is expected to continue to evolve as more experience and confidence are accrued in the operating characteristics of the methods and interpretability of the associated results.

BIBLIOGRAPHY

Alemayehu, D., Chen, Y., Markatou, M. (2018) A comparative study of subgroup identification methods for differential treatment effect: Performance metrics and recommendations. *Statistical Methods in Medical Research.* 27(12): 3658–3678.

Akacha, M., Bretz, F., Ohlssen, D., Rosenkranz, G., Schmidli, H. (2017) Estimands and their role in clinical trials. *Statistics in Biopharmaceutical Research.* 9(3): 268–271.

Alosh, M., Bretz, F., Huque, M. (2014) Advanced multiplicity adjustment methods in clinical trials. *Statistics in Medicine.* 33: 693–713.

Andridge, R. R., Little, R. J. A. (2010) A review of hot deck imputation for survey nonresponse. *International Statistical Review.* 78: 40–64; *Annals of Internal Medicine.* 147: 573–577. (Erratum in: *Annals of Internal Medicine.* 148: 168).

Angelis, A., Kanavos, P. (2017) Multiple criteria decision analysis (MCDA) for evaluating new medicines in health technology assessment and beyond: The advance value framework. *Social Science & Medicine.* 188: 137–156.

Anthenelli, R. M. (2016) Neuropsychiatric safety and efficacy of varenicline, bupropion, and nicotine patch in smokers with and without psychiatric disorders (EAGLES): A double-blind, randomized, placebo-controlled clinical trial. *The Lancet.* 387(10037): P2507–2520.

Bauer, P., Kohne, K. (1994) Evaluation of experiments with adaptive interim analyses. *Biometrics.* December 1. 50(4): 1029–1041.

Benjamini, Y., Hochberg, Y. (1995) Controlling the false discovery rate: A practical and powerful approach to multiple testing. *Journal of the Royal Statistical Society B.* 57(1): 289–300.

Berger, V. W. (2004) Does the Prentice criterion validate surrogate endpoints? Statistics in Medicine. 23: 1571–1578

Berry, S. M. Broglio, K. R., Groshen, S. (2013) Bayesian hierarchical modeling of patient subpopulations: Efficient designs of Phase II oncology clinical trials. *Clinical Trials*. 10: 720–734.

Braun, T. M., Wang, S. (2010) A hierarchical Bayesian design for phase I trials of novel combinations of cancer therapeutic agents. *Biometrics*. 66: 805–812.

Breiman, L., Friedman, J. H., Olshen, R. A., Stone, C. J. (1984) *Classification and Regression Trees*. Monterey: Wadsworth & Brooks/Cole Advanced Books & Software. ISBN 978-0-412-04841-8.

Buyse, M., Molenberghs, M., Paoletti, X., Oba, K., Alonso, A., Van der Elst, W., Burzykowski, T. (2015) Statistical evaluation of surrogate endpoints with examples from cancer clinical trials. *Biometrical Journal*. 58(1): 104–132.

Centre for Innovation in Regulatory Science. (2012) Workshop synopsis: Building the benefit-risk toolbox: Are there enough common elements across the different methodologies to enable a consensus on a scientifically acceptable framework for making benefit-risk decisions? Available online at: http://cirsci.org/publications/CIRS_June_2012_Workshop_Synopsis.pdf (accessed June 7, 2019).

Chau, C. H., Rixe, O., McLeod, H., Figg, W. D. (2008) Validation of analytic methods for biomarkers used in drug development. *Clinical Cancer Research*. 14(19), October 1: 5967–5976.

Chen, C., Li, X. N., Yuan, S., Antonijevic, z., Kalamegham, R., Beckman, R. A. (2016) Statistical design and considerations of a phase 3 basket trial for simultaneous investigation of multiple tumor types in one study. *Statistics in Biopharmaceutical Research*. 8: 248–257.

Chen, Y. H., DeMets, D. L., Lan, K. K. (2004) Increasing the sample size when the unblinded interim result is promising. *Statistics in Medicine*. 23: 1023–1038.

Chow, S.-C., Chang, M., Pong, A. (2005) Statistical consideration of adaptive methods in clinical development. *Journal of Biopharmaceutical Statistics*. 15: 575–591.

Chung, S. C., Schulz, M. (2007) Bayesian designs for clinical trials in early drug development. *Journal of Clinical Research Best Practices*. 3: 1–5.

Cui, L., Hung, H. M., Wang S. J. (1999) Modification of sample size in group sequential 1277 clinical trials, *Biometrics*. 55(3), September 1: 853–857.

Cunanan, K. M., Shen, R., Iasonos, A. et al. (2017) An efficient basket trial design. *Statistics in Medicine*. 36: 1568–1579.

Denne, J. S. (2001) Sample size recalculation using conditional power. *Statistics in Medicine*. 1285 20(17–18), September 15: 2645–2660.

DeRubeis, R. J., Cohen, Z. D., Forand, N. R., Fournier, J. C., Gelfand, A., Lorenzo-Luaces, L. (2014) The personalized advantage index: Translating research on prediction into individualized treatment recommendations. *PLoS ONE*. 9(1): Article ID e83875.

Diggle, P., Kenward, M. G. (1994) Informative drop-out in longitudinal data analysis (with discussion). *Applied Statistics*. 43: 49–93.

Dmitrienko, A., D'Agostino, R. B. (2013) Tutorial in biostatistics: Traditional multiplicity adjustment methods in clinical trials. *Statistics in Medicine*. 32: 5172–5218.

Dmitrienko, A., D'Agostino, R. B., Huque, M. F. (2013) Key multiplicity issues in clinical drug development. *Statistics in Medicine*. 32: 1079–1111.

Dmitrienko, A., Tamhane, A. C., Bretz, F. (editors) (2009) *Multiple Testing Problems in Pharmaceutical Statistics*. New York: Chapman and Hall/CRC Press.

Ellenberg, S., Fleming, T., DeMets, D. (2002) *Data Monitoring Committees in Clinical Trials: A Practical Perspective*. Chichester: John Wiley & Sons.

EQUATOR Network (2017) Enhancing the quality and transparency of health research. www.equator-network.org (accessed May 11, 2017).

European Medicines Agency (2010a) Benefit-risk methodology project. Work package 2 report: Applicability of current tools and processes for regulatory benefit-risk assessment. Available online at: www.ema.europa.eu/docs/en_GB/document_library/Report/2010/10/WC500097750.pdf (accessed June 15, 2019).

European Medicines Agency (2010b) Guidelines on missing data in confirmatory clinical trials. July 2, (accessed January 29, 2019). Available from: www.ema.europa.eu/docs/en_GB/document./WC500096793.pdf.

European Medicines Agency (2011) Implementing the European Medicines Agency's roadmap to 2015: The agency's contribution to science, medicines, health. Available online at: www.ema.europa.eu/docs/en_GB/document_library/Other/2011/10/WC500115960.pdf (accessed December 16, 2014).

European Medicinal Agency (2015). Guidance document on the content of the Rapporteur day 80 critical assessment report. Overview and lists of question. EMA/90842/2015. Available from http://www.ema.europa.eu/docs/en_GB/document_library/Regulatory_and_procedural_guideline/2009/10/WC500004800.pdf

European Medicines Agency (EMA) (2017a) Essential considerations for successful qualification of novel methodologies. (accessed June 7, 2019). www.ema.europa.eu/en/documents/other/essential-considerations-successful-qualification-novel-methodologies_en.pdf.

European Medicines Agency (2017b) Guideline on multiplicity issues in clinical trials. Available online at: www.ema.europa.eu/en/documents/scientific-guideline/draft-guideline-multiplicity-issues-clinical-trials_en.pdf.

European Medicines Agency (2019) Investigation of subgroups in confirmatory clinical trials European Medicine Agency; Committee for Medicinal Products for Human Use (CHMP). January 2019.

European Network for Health Technology Assessment (EUnetHTA) (2013) Endpoints used in REA of pharmaceuticals: surrogate endpoints. (accessed June 7, 2018). www.eunethta.eu/wp-content/uploads/2018/01/Surrogate-Endpoints.pdf.

FDA-NIH Biomarker Working Group (2016) BEST (Biomarkers, Endpoints, and other Tools) Resource [Internet]. Silver Spring (MD): Food and Drug Administration (US); Glossary. January 28, 2016 [Updated May 2, 2018]. Available from: www.ncbi.nlm.nih.gov/books/NBK338448/ Co-published by National Institutes of Health (US), Bethesda (MD).

Finkelstein, D. M., Schoenfeld, D. A. (1999) Combining mortality and longitudinal measures in clinical trials. *Statistics in Medicine.* 18(11): 1341–1354.

Fitzmaurice, G. M., Lipsitz, S. R., Molenberghs, G. et al. (2000) Bias in estimating association parameters for longitudinal binary responses with drop-outs. *Biometrics.* 56(1): 528–536.

Fleming, T. (2005) Surrogate endpoints and FDA's accelerated approval process. *Health Affairs.* 24(1): 67–78.

Food and Drug Administration (2010) Guidance for industry and FDA staff: Guidance for the use of Bayesian statistics in medical device clinical trials. (accessed on December 3, 2018). Available from: www.fda.gov/ucm/groups/fdagovpublic/@fdagov-meddev-gen/documents/document/ucm071121.pdf

Food Drug Administration (2013) Structured approach to benefit-risk assessment in drug regulatory decision-making. Draft DPUFA V implementation plan. Fiscal years 2013017. Available online at: www.fda.gov/downloads/ForIndustry/UserFees/PrescriptionDrugUserFee/UCM329758.pdf (accessed June 7, 2019).

Food and Drug Administration (2016) Non-inferiority clinical trials to establish effectiveness guidance for industry. U.S. Department of Health and Human Services: Center for Drug Evaluation and Research (CDER), Center for Biologics Evaluation and Research (CBER): November 2016.

Food and Drug Administration (2017a) Evaluation and reporting of age-, race-, and ethnicity-specific data in medical device clinical studies. Guidance for industry and Food and Drug Administration staff. September.

Food and Drug Administration (2017b) Multiple endpoints in clinical trials: Guidance for industry. (U.S. Department of Health and Human Services Food and Drug Administration, January 2017).

www.fda.gov/downloads/drugs/guidancecomplianceregulatoryinformation/guidances/ucm536750.pdf.

Food and Drug Administration (2017c) The FDA's drug review process: Ensuring drugs are safe and effective.

www.fda.gov/drugs/resourcesforyou/consumers/ucm143534.htm (accessed May 11, 2017).

Food and Drug Administration (2018a) CDER biomarker qualification program (BQP). (accessed June 7, 2018). www.fda.gov/drugs/drug-development-tool-qualification-programs/cder-biomarker-qualification-program.

Food and Drug Administration (2018b) Medical product communications that are consistent with the FDA-required labeling questions and answers; Guidance for industry. US Department of Health and Human Services; Food and Drug Administration. June 2018.

Food and Drug Administration (2019) Enrichment strategies for clinical trials to support demonstration of effectiveness of human drugs and biological products. (accessed June 7, 2019). www.fda.gov/media/121320/download.

Foster, J. C., Taylor, J. M. C., Ruberg, S. J. (2011) Subgroup identification from randomized clinical trial data. *Statistics in Medicine*. 30: 2867–2880.

Freedman, L. S. Graubard, B. I., Schatzkin, A. et al. (1992) Statistical validation of intermediate endpoints for chronic disease. *Statistics in Medicine*. 11: 167–178.

Freidlin B., Korn, E. L. (2013) Borrowing information across subgroups in phase II trials: Is it useful? *Clinical Cancer Research*. 19: 1326–1334.

Gaffney, M. (2016) Statistical issues in the design, conduct and analysis of two large safety studies. *Clinical Trials*. 13(5): 513–518. Published online: June, 2016; Issue published: October 2016.

Gaffney, M.,Ware, J. H. (2017) An evaluation of increasing sample size based on conditional power. *Journal of Biopharmaceutical Statistics*. 27(5): 797–808

Gail, M., Simon, R. (1985) Testing for qualitative interactions between treatment effects and patient subsets. *Biometrics*. 41: 361–372.

Gelfand, A. E., Smith, A. F. M. (1990) Sampling-based approaches to calculating marginal densities. *Journal of the American Statistical Association*. 85: 398–409.

Ghosh, P., Liu, L., Senchaudhuri, P., Gao, P., Mehta, C. (2017) Design and monitoring of multi-arm multi-stage clinical trials. *Biometrics*. 73: 1289–1299.

Greco, T., Biondi-Zoccai, G., Saleh, O., Pasin, L., Cabrini, L., Zangrillo, A., Landoni, G. (2015) The attractiveness of network meta-analysis: A comprehensive systematic and narrative review. *Heart, Lung and Vessels*, 7(2): 133–142.

Guo, J. J., Pandey, S., Doyle, J., Bian, B., Lis, Y., Raisch, D. W. (2010) A review of quantitative risk-benefit methodologies for assessing drug safety and efficacy-report of the ISPOR risk-benefit management working group. *Value in Health*. 13(5), August: 657–666.

Hastie, T., Tibshirani, R., Friedman, J. (2009) *The Elements of Statistical Learning: Data Mining, Inference and Prediction*. New York: Springer.

Hobbs, B. P., Chen, N., Lee, J. J. (2016) Controlled multi-arm platform design using predictive probability. *Statistical Methods in Medical Research.* 27: 65–78.

Hughes, D., Waddingham, E., Mt-Isa, S., Goginsky, A., Chan, E., Downey, G. F. et al. (2016) Recommendations for benefit-risk assessment methodologies and visual representations. *Pharmacoepidemiology and Drug Safety.* 25: 251–262.

Huque, M. F., Dmitrienko, A., D'Agostino, R. B. (2013) Multiplicity issues in clinical trials with multiple objectives. *Statistics in Biopharmaceutical Research.* 5: 321–337.

Ibrahim, J. G., Molenberghs, G. (2009) Missing data methods in longitudinal studies: A review. *Test (Madr).* 18(1): 1–43.

Ibrahim, J. G., Chen, M. H., Gwon, Y., Chen, F. (2015) The power prior: Theory and applications. *Statistics in Medicine.* 34(28): 3724–3749.

International Conference on Harmonization Guidance for Industry E10 (2001) Choice of control group and related issues in clinical trials. U.S. Department of Health and Human Services, Food and Drug Administration, Center for Drug Evaluation and Research (CDER), Center for Biologics Evaluation and Research (CBER). May 2001.

International Conference on Harmonisation ICH E9 (1999) Expert working group. Statistical principles for clinical trials: ICH harmonized tripartite guideline. Statistics in Medicine. 18: 1905–1942.

International Conference on Harmonisation ICH E9 (R1) (2017) Addendum on estimands and sensitivity analysis in clinical trials to the guideline on statistical principles for clinical trials EMA/CHMP/ICH/436221/2017. Available at: www.ema.europa.eu/documents/scientific-guideline/draft-ich-e9-r1-addendum-estimands-sensitivity-analysis-clinical-trials-guideline-statistical_en.pdf.

International Conference on Harmonisation of Technical Requirements for Registration of Pharmaceuticals for Human Use (1998) ICH harmonised tripartite guideline E9: Statistical principles for clinical trials.

International Conference on Harmonisation of Technical Requirements for Registration of Pharmaceuticals for Human Use (June 2016) Revision of M4E guideline on enhancing the format and structure of benefit-risk information in ICH efficacy. Retrieved from www.ich.org/fileadmin/Public_Web_Site/ICH_Products/CTD/M4E_R2_Efficacy/M4E_R2__Step_4.pdf.

Jennison, C. Turnbull, B. W. (1999) *Group Sequential Methods with Applications to Clinical Trials.* New York: CRC Press. September 15.

Kaizer, A. M., Hobbs, B. P., Koopmeiners, J. S. (2018) A multi-source adaptive platform design for testing sequential combinatorial therapeutic strategies. *Biometrics.* 74(3): 1082–1094. 10.1111/biom.12841

Keeney, R. L., Raiffa, H. (1976) *Decision with Multiple Objectives: Preferences and Value Tradeoffs.* New York: John Wiley & Sons.

Kenward, M. G. (1998) Selection models for repeated measurements with non-random dropout: An illustration of sensitivity. *Statistics in Medicine*. 17(23), December 15: 2723–2732.

Kimani, P. K., Glimm, E., Maurer, W., Hutton, J. L., Stallard, N. (2012) Practical guidelines for adaptive seamless phase II/III clinical trials that use Bayesian methods. *Statistics in Medicine*. 31(19): 2068–2085.

Korn, E. L., Freidlin, B. (2011) Outcome-adaptive randomization: Is it useful? Journal of *Clinical Oncology*. 29: 771–776.

Kwok, H., Lewis, R. J. (2011) Bayesian hierarchical modeling and the integration of heterogeneous information on the effectiveness of cardiovascular therapies. *Circulation: Cardiovascular Quality and Outcomes*. 4: 657–666.

Lan, K. K. G., DeMets, D. L. (1983) Discrete sequential boundaries for clinical trials. *Biometrika*. 70(3): 659–663.

LaVange, L. M., Permutt, T. (2016) A regulatory perspective on missing data in the aftermath of the NRC report. *Statistics in Medicine*. 35: 2853–2864.

Lavori, P. W., Dawson, R., Shera, D. (1995) A multiple imputation strategy for clinical trials with truncation of patient data. *Statistics in Medicine*. 14: 1913–1925.

Le Tourneau, C., Lee, J. J., Siu, L. L. (2009) Dose escalation methods in phase I cancer clinical 1326 trials. *Journal of the National Cancer Institute*. 101(10), May 20: 708–720.

LeBlanc M., Rankin, C., Crowley, J. (2009) Multiple histology phase II trials. *Clinical Cancer Research*. 15: 4256–4262.

Lee, C. Y. Y., Wand, M. P. (2015) Variational methods for fitting complex Bayesian mixed effects models to health data statistics in medicine. *Statistics in Medicine*. 35: 165–188.

Levin, G. P., Emerson, S. C., Emerson, S. S. (2013) Adaptive clinical trial designs with pre-specified rules for modifying the sample size: Understanding efficient types of adaptation. *Statistics in Medicine*. 32(8): 1259–1275; discussion 1280–1282. DOI: 10.1002/sim.5662.

Levitan, B. (2012) Evaluating benefit–risk during and beyond drug development: An industry view. *Regulatory Rapporteur*. 9: 10–15.

Li, K., Yuan, S. S., Wang, W., Wan, S. S., Ceesay, P., Heyse, J. F., Mt-Isa, S., Luo, S. (2018) Periodic benefit-risk assessment using Bayesian stochastic multi-criteria acceptability analysis. *Contemporary Clinical Trials*. 67, April: 100–108.

Little, R. J. A., JSTOR (1995) Modeling the drop-out mechanism in repeated-measures studies. *Journal of American Statistical Association*. 90: 1113–1121.

Little, R. J., Wang, Y. (1996) Pattern-mixture models for multivariate incomplete data with covariates. Biometrics. 52(1): 98–111.

Little, R. J., D'Agostino, R., Cohen, M. L. et al. (2012) The prevention and treatment of missing data in clinical trials. *New England Journal of Medicine*. 367: 1355–1360.

Liu, R., Liu, Z., Ghadessi, M., Vonk, R. (2017) Increasing the efficiency of oncology basket trials using a Bayesian approach. *Contemporary Clinical Trials.* 63: 67–72.

Liublinska, V., Rubin, D. B. (2014) Sensitivity analysis for a partially missing binary outcome in a two-arm randomized clinical trial. *Statistics in Medicine.* 33(24): 4170–4185.

Liu-Seifert, H., Zhang, S., D'Souza, D., Skljarevski, V. (2010) A closer look at the baseline-observation-carried-forward (BOCF). *Patient Prefer Adherence.* 4: 11–16.

Lu, W., Zhang, H. H., Zeng, D. (2013) Variable selection for optimal treatment decision. *Statistical Methods in Medical Research.* 22: 493–504.

Lunn, D., Spiegelhalter, D., Thomas, A., Best, N. (2009) The BUGS project: Evolution, critique and future directions. *Statistics in Medicine.* 28: 3049–3067.

Madigan, D., Ryan, P., Simpson, S. E., Zorych, I. (2010) Bayesian methods in pharmacovigilance (with discussion). In: Bernardo, J. M., Bayarri, M. J., Berger, J. O., Dawid, A. P., Heckerman, D., Smith, A. F. M., West, M., editors. *Bayesian Statistics* 9. New York: Oxford University Press: 421–438.

Mallinckrodt, C. H., Sanger, T. M., Dubé, S., DeBrota, D. J., Molenberghs, G., Carroll, R. J., Potter, W. Z., Tollefson, G. D. (2003) Assessing and interpreting treatment effects in longitudinal clinical trials with missing data. *Biological Psychiatry.* 53(8): 754–760.

Mauer, M., Collette, L., Bogaerts, J. (2012) European Organisation for Research and Treatment of Cancer (EORTC) Statistics Department. Adaptive designs at European Organisation for Research and Treatment of Cancer (EORTC) with a focus on adaptive sample size re-estimation based on interim-effect size. *European Journal of Cancer.* 48: 1386–1391.

Matsui, S. (2013) Genomic biomarkers for personalized medicine: Development and validation in clinical studies. *Computational and Mathematical Methods in Medicine.* 2013: 865980. DOI: 10.1155/2013/865980.

Mehta, C. R., Pocock, S. J. (2011) Adaptive increase in sample size when interim results are promising: A practical guide with examples. *Statistics in Medicine.* 30(28): 3267–3284.

Mentz, R. J., Hernandez, A. F., Berdan, L. G. et al. (2016) Good clinical practice guidance and pragmatic clinical trials: Balancing the best of both worlds. *Circulation.* 133: 872–880.

Mott, D. J. (2018) Incorporating quantitative patient preference data into healthcare decision making processes: Is HTA falling behind? *Patient.* 11: 249–252.

Murad, M. H., Asi, N., Alsawas, M. et al. (2016) New evidence pyramid. *Evidence Based Medicine.* 21: 125–127.

National Cancer Institute (2014) Targeted cancer therapies. National Cancer Institute website. www.cancer.gov/about-cancer/treatment/types/targeted-therapies/targeted-therapies-fact-sheet. Updated April 25, 2014. (accessed December 13, 2016).

National Research Council (2010) *The Prevention and Treatment of Missing Data in Clinical Trials*. Washington DC: The National Academies Press, Panel on Handling Missing Data in Clinical Trials. Committee on National Statistics, Division of Behavioral and Social Sciences and Education.

Nissen, S. E. (2016) Cardiovascular safety of Celecoxib, Naproxen, or Ibuprofen for arthritis. *New England Journal of Medicine*. 10(1056): 2519–2529.

O'Brien, P. C., Fleming, T. R. (1979) A multiple testing procedure for clinical trials. *Biometrics*. September 1. 35(3): 549–556.

O'Neill, R. T., Temple, R. (2012) The prevention and treatment of missing data in clinical trials: An FDA perspective on the importance of dealing with it. *Clinical Pharmacology & Therapeutics*. 9(3): 550–554.

O'Quigley, J., Pepe, M., Fisher, L. (1990) Continual reassessment method: A practical design for phase 1 clinical trials in cancer. *Biometrics*. 46: 43–48.

Paoletti, X., Oba, K., Bang, Y. J. et al. (2013) Progression-free survival as a surrogate for overall survival in advanced/recurrent gastric cancer trials: A meta-analysis. *Journal of National Cancer Institute*. 105(21): 1667–1670.

Pennello, G., Thompson, L. (2008) Experience with reviewing Bayesian medical device trials. *Journal of Biopharmaceutical Statistics*, 18(1): 81–115.

Pocock, S. J. (1977) Group sequential methods in the design and analysis of clinical trials. *Biometrika*. 64(2): 191–199.

Pocock, S. J., Simon, R. (1975) Sequential treatment assignment with balancing for prognostic factors in the controlled clinical trial. *Biometrics*. 31(1), March 1: 103–115.

Pocock, S. J., Ariti, C. A., Collier, T. J., Wang, D. (2012) The win ratio: A new approach to the analysis of composite endpoints in clinical trials based on clinical priorities. *European Heart Journal*. 33(2): 176–182.

Pocock, S. J., Assmann, S. E., Enos, L. E., Kasten, L. E. (2002) Subgroup analysis, covariate adjustment and baseline comparisons in clinical trial reporting: Current practice and problems. *Statistics in Medicine*. 21: 2917–2930.

Preisser J. S., Lohman, K. K., Rathouz, P. J. (2002) Performance of weighted estimating equations for longitudinal binary data with drop-outs missing at random. Statistics in Medicine. 21: 3035–3054.

Prentice, R. L. (1989) Surrogate endpoints in clinical trials: Definitions and operational criteria. *Statistics in Medicine*. 8: 431–440.

Proschan, M. A., Hunsberger, S. A. (1995) Designed extension of studies based on conditional power. *Biometrics*. December 1. 51(4): 1315–1324.

Proschan, M. A., Waclawiw, M. A. (2000) Practical guidelines for multiplicity adjustment in clinical trials. *Controlled Clinical Trials*. 21: 527–539.

Robins, J. M., Rotnitzky, A., Zhao, L. P. (1995) Analysis of semiparametric regression models for repeated outcomes in the presence of missing data. *Journal of the American Statistical Association*. 90(429): 106–121.

Rosenbaum, P. R., Rubin, D. B. (1983) The central role of the propensity score in observational studies for causal effects. *Biometrika*. 70(1): 41–55.

Rosenberger, W. F. (1999) Randomized play-the-winner clinical trials: Review and recommendations. *Controlled Clinical Trials*. 20: 328–342.

Rubin D. B. (1987) *Multiple Imputation for Nonresponse in Surveys*. New York: John Wiley & Sons.

Saint-Hilary, G., Cadour, S., Robert, V., Gasparini, M. (2017) A simple way to unify multicriteria decision analysis (MCDA) and stochastic multicriteria acceptability analysis (SMAA) using a Dirichlet distribution in benefit–risk assessment. *Biometrical Journal*. 59(3), May 1: 567–578.

Schafer, J. L. (1997) *Analysis of Incomplete Multivariate Data*. New York: Chapman and Hall.

Schmidli, H., Bretz, F., Racine-Poon, A. (2007) Bayesian predictive power for interim adaptation in seamless phase II/III trials where the endpoint is survival up to some specified timepoint. *Statistics in Medicine*. 26: 4925–4938.

Schoenfeld, D. A. (1983) Sample-size formula for the proportional-hazards regression model. *Biometrics*. 39: 499–503.

Schwartz, D., Lellouch, J. (1967) Explanatory and pragmatic attitudes in therapeutical trials. *Journal of Chronic Diseases*. 20: 637–648.

Simon, R. (1989) Optimal two-stage designs for phase II clinical trials. *Controlled Clinical Trials*. 10(1): 1–10.

Simon, R. (2010) Clinical trial designs for evaluating the medical utility of prognostic and predictive biomarkers in oncology. *Personalised Medicine*. 7(1), January 1: 33–47.

Simon, R. (2017a) Critical review of umbrella, basket, and platform designs for oncology clinical trials. *Clinical Pharmacology & Therapeutics*. 102(6), December: 934.

Simon, R. (2017b) New designs for basket clinical trials in oncology. *Journal of Biopharmaceutical Statistics*. 28: 245–255.

Simon, R., Geyer, S., Subramanian, J., Roychowdhury, S. (2016) The Bayesian basket design for genomic variant-driven phase II clinical trials. *Seminars in Oncology*. 43: 13–18.

Speed, T. (2003) *Statistical Analysis of Gene Expression Microarray Data*. Boca Raton: Chapman and Hall, CRC Press.

Spiegelhalter, D. J., Myles, J. P., Jones, D. R., Abrams, K. R. (2000) Bayesian methods in health technology assessment: A review. *Health Technology Assessment*. 4: 1–130.

Stallard, N., Todd, S. (2010) Seamless phase II/III design. *Statistical Methods in Medical Research.* 20(6): 623–634.

Storey, J. D. Tibshirani, R. (2003) Statistical significance for genome-wide studies. *Proceedings of the National Academy of Sciences.* 100: 9440–9445.

Su, X., Tsai, C-L., Wang, H., Nickerson, D. M., Li, B. (2009) Subgroup analysis via recursive partitioning. *Journal of Machine Learning Research.* 10: 141–158.

Tanniou, J., van der Tweel, I., Teerenstra, S., Roes, K. C. B. (2016) Subgroup analyses in confirmatory clinical trials: Time to be specific about their purposes. *BMC Medical Research Methodology.* BMC series. 16: 20.

Tervonen, T., van Valkenhoef, G., Buskens, E., Hillege, H. L., Postmus, D. A. (2011) Stochastic multicriteria model for evidence-based decision making in drug benefit-risk analysis. *Statistics in Medicine.* 30: 1419–1428.

Thokala, P., Devlin, N., Marsh, K. et al. (2016) Multiple criteria decision analysis for health care decision making – an introduction: Report 1 of the ISPOR MCDA Emerging Good Practices Task Force. *Value in Health.* 19(1): 1–13.

Thall, P. F. Wathen, J. K., Bekele, B. N. et al. (2003) Hierarchical Bayesian approaches to phase II trials in diseases with multiple subtypes. *Statistics in Medicine.* 22: 763–780.

Thall, P. F., Wathen, J. K. (2007) Practical Bayesian adaptive randomisation in clinical trials. *European Journal of Cancer.* 43: 859–866.

US Department of Health and Human Services Food and Drug Administration, Center for Drug Evaluation and Research (CDER), Center for Biologics Evaluation and Research (CBER). Guidance for Industry: (2018a) Adaptive design clinical trials for drugs and biologics. Draft Guidance. September.

US Department of Health and Human Services Food and Drug Administration, Center for Drug Evaluation and Research (CDER), Center for Biologics Evaluation and Research (CBER). Guidance for Industry: (2018b) Expansion cohorts: Use in first-in-human clinical trials to expedite development of oncology drugs and biologics. Draft Guidance. September.

Van Buuren, S. (2007) Multiple imputation of discrete and continuous data by fully conditional specification. *Statistical Methods in Medical Research.* 16: 219–242.

Vandenbroucke, J. P., von Elm, E., Altman, D. G. et al. (2007) STROBE initiative. Strengthening the reporting of observational studies in epidemiology (STROBE): Explanation and elaboration.

van Valkenhoef, G., Tervonen, T., Zwinkels, T., Brock, B., Hillege, H. (2013) ADDIS: A decision support system for evidence-based medicine. *Decision Support Systems.* 55: 459–475. DOI: 10.1016/j.dss.2012.10.005.

Viele, K., Berry, S., Neuenschwander, B., Amzal, B., Chen, F., Enas, N., Hobbs, B., Ibrahim, J. G., Kinnersley, N., Lindborg, S., Micallef, S., Roychoudhury, S., Thompson, L. (2014) Use of historical control data for assessing treatment effects in clinical trials. *Pharmaceutical Statistics*. 13(1): 41–54. https://doi.org/10.1002/pst.1589.

Waddingham, E., Mt-Isa, S., Nixon, R., Ashby, D. (2016) A Bayesian approach to probabilistic sensitivity analysis in structured benefit-risk assessment. *Biometrical Journal*. 58(1), January 1: 28–42.

Wang, R., Lagakos, S. W., Ware, J. H., Hunter, D. J., Drazen, J. M. (2007) Statistics in medicine – Reporting of subgroup analyses in clinical trials. *New England Journal of Medicine*. 357: 2189–2194.

Wang, Y., Taylor, J. M. G. (2003) A measure of the proportion of treatment effect explained by a surrogate marker. *Biometrics*. 58: 803–812.

Wasserstein, R. L., Lazar, N. A. (2016) The ASA's statement on p-values: Context, process, and purpose. *The American Statistician*. 70: 129–133.

Wassmer, G., Brannath, W. (2016) *Group Sequential and Confirmatory Adaptive Designs in Clinical Trials*. Springer series in pharmaceutical statistics. New York: Springer.

Wittes, J., Brittain, E. (1990) The role of internal pilot studies in increasing the efficiency of clinical trials. *Statistics in Medicine*. 9: 65–72.

Wu, M. C., Bailey, K. R. (1989) Estimation and comparison of changes in the presence of informative right censoring: Conditional linear model. *Biometrics*. 45: 939–955.

Yuan, S. S., Chen, A., Chen, C. et al. (2016) On group sequential enrichment design for basket trial. *Statistics in Biopharmaceutical Research*. 8: 293–306.

Zellner, A. (1988) Optimal information processing and Bayes' theorem (with discussion). *The American Statistician*. 42: 278–284.

Zikopoulos, P. C., Eaton, C., deRoos, D. et al. (2012) *Understanding Big Data: Analytics for Enterprise Class Hadoop and Streaming Data*. New York McGraw Hill. www.ibm.com/developerworks/vn/library/contest/dw-freebooks/Tim_Hieu_Big_Data/Understanding_BigData.PDF (accessed May 11, 2017).

CHAPTER 3

Statistical Engagement in Regulatory Interactions

3.1 INTRODUCTION

It is indisputable that the discipline of statistics is quite important in many interactions between pharmaceutical companies and regulatory agencies regarding drug development, drug approval, and drug promotion (Lewi 2005). This importance may be due to the statistical methods applied to the raw data and/or the interpretation of the analyzed results (Marquardt 1987). This is true whether the application of statistics concerns randomized trials or observational databases for real-world evidence and cost-effectiveness evaluation. This points to a prominent role of the statistician within these activities. This role is often recognized within the pharmaceutical company and among regulatory agencies, as can be inferred from the various guidance documents and reflection papers issued by the US Food and Drug Administration (FDA), the European Medicines Agency (EMA), and the International Council for Harmonization of Technical Requirements for Pharmaceuticals for Human Use (ICH).

The design of studies is typically a joint activity between the statistician and the clinician, but the analytical methods are almost exclusively the provenance of the statistician. The interpretation of the results is also strongly influenced by the methods used in the analysis and the conclusions of the statistician. This prominent role of the statistician does not always extend to a strategic role within the company or to a broader representative role in regulatory interaction. Ideally, the statistician should think strategically about the totality of the data and thereby have a wider role than a purely statistical one internally and in regulatory interaction (Rockhold 2009). This is less about the definition of roles or overcoming barriers or the need to sell the statistical profession (Grieve 2002). Those are past battles that have been largely won. This is more about behaviors and knowing when to insert oneself into the game (Emir et al. 2013; Grieve 2005; Unwin 2007). Specific areas of statistical activity are examined in this chapter with the focus on highlighting behaviors to enhance the strategic and representative roles of the statistician in regulatory and other external interactions.

3.2 INTERNAL BEHAVIORS

The statistician's ability to be influential directly in regulatory interactions must first be established and recognized within the pharmaceutical company itself. Thus, the behaviors begin at home. Even the prominent internal role of the statistician in the design, analysis, and interpretation of study results is often not enough to consider the statistician as more than a supportive role in direct interaction with regulators. Access to the process as a strategic player often happens as a result of behaviors and successes on past projects. Statisticians should look to make presentations within the pharmaceutical company to non-statistics groups (e.g., regulatory, clinical, marketing, or outcomes research) relating statistical methods and principles to regulatory topics. For example, the concept of "estimands" is a statistical issue with a strong regulatory impact. Statisticians should take the initiative on explaining this concept and its application to clinical trial analysis and interpretation. Thus, when the inevitable regulatory issue of estimands arises in the design and/or analysis of clinical trials, the statistician should be perceived as the critical person to represent the company in the interaction with regulators.

Statisticians should also be well-versed in applicable regulations and review and comment on draft regulatory guidance. For example, in June 2018 the US FDA issued a guidance for industry titled, "Medical product communications that are consistent with the FDA-required labeling" (FDA 2018). This guidance recognized that sponsors have additional information about approved uses of their products that is consistent with the label, and communication of this information to patients and prescribers is helpful. The guidance deals with how FDA evaluates consistency of a product communication with the product's labeling and gives general recommendations for conveying information in a truthful and non-misleading way. While not overtly statistical in nature, the guidance does rely on the concept of "false and misleading." To avoid being false and misleading there should be scientifically appropriate and statistically sound support for the promotional communication. The guidance points out that findings or the conclusions that can be drawn from supportive data should not be overstated. The communication requires proper contextual language including "limitations of the strength of evidence." The statistician is the most appropriate person to make sure these criteria are satisfied, but regulatory and marketing groups within a pharmaceutical company may not recognize this. However, a statistician who takes the initiative to summarize the guidance and what communications may or may not satisfy the "false and misleading" criterion from a statistical perspective will enhance his/her strategic value.

Some external activities can also lead to a bigger strategic role in regulatory interaction. Publications on statistical methodology, applied to clinical trials or any other field in general, is one such activity. Making presentations at scientific meetings and serving on joint regulatory and industry working groups are others. However, because these activities may not be fully known or appreciated by senior management and do not include direct interaction between the project teams and the statistician, the influence of external activities may be limited. The direct, internal strategic activities are more effective in establishing the strategic role of the statistician in regulatory interaction. As discussed in the next section, with the extensive use of external Data-Monitoring Committees on important clinical trials, the role of the independent statistician in such committees offers another way to increase the strategic role of the statistician within the pharmaceutical company.

3.3 DATA MONITORING COMMITTEE

Data Monitoring Committees (DMCs) are utilized by pharmaceutical companies to monitor unblinded the accumulating data in a clinical trial (Ellenberg et al. 2002; Herson 2009). The purpose of a DMC is to ensure the safety of the participants in the trial and to ensure the quality and integrity of the trial. The DMC is usually comprised of outside experts in the disease area, clinical trial methodology, and statistics (DeMets et al. 2006).

The trials that require DMCs often deal with mortality/morbidity endpoints and are critical to the regulatory success of the treatment. Thus, these trials have high visibility and importance for the sponsor and for the external medical and regulatory environments. There are different DMC models acceptable to regulatory authorities (FDA 2006). It is not the purpose here to contrast the strengths and weaknesses of the various models. However, one model is to have the sponsor serve as the data coordinating center (DCC), i.e., the sponsor is responsible for data collection, establishing the database, and preparing the periodic review tables for the DMC. In this model the independent statistician, i.e., the statistician responsible for the preparation of review tables and presentation of data at the closed DMC meeting, comes from the sponsor. Thus, this is a critical role with high visibility that can lead to a greater strategic and representative role of the statistician in regulatory interaction.

The responsibilities of the independent statistician, whether employed by the sponsor or has no direct affiliation with it, include detailed knowledge of the review tables and often to present these tables to DMC members in the closed meeting. To do this effectively, the independent statistician should be well-versed in the study protocol and statistical analysis plan as well as the review tables. While the independent statistician is not typically a member of the DMC, he or she may be asked to guide the DMC discussion of the tables and should be alert to any misinterpretation of the table contents. In short, a good independent statistician facilitates the work of the DMC, while ensuring that the integrity of the study is preserved. By the end of the study the independent statistician will be knowledgeable about all aspects of the study conduct and analysis. In addition, the independent-statistician role allows the statistician to interact with internal study leadership and external members of the DMC. This positions the statistician to take on a strategic role in any ensuing regulatory interaction regarding this study and drug.

From a methodological point of view, the role of the statistician extends to ensuring that appropriate measures are in place to protect against Type I error inflation as well as any potential bias that may arise as a consequence of the activities of the DMC. For example, even when the mandate of a DMC is to evaluate safety, and not to monitor the primary endpoint to recommend study termination for futility or evidence of efficacy, there may be a need to look at unblinded efficacy data to assess the relative risks and benefits of the drug to guide the DMC recommendations. In such cases, the statistician should formulate effective justifications about whether Type I error adjustment is necessary or not (see, e.g., EMA 2005).

3.4 REGULATORY MEETINGS AND ADVISORY COMMITTEE MEETINGS

This section will deal with the strategic role of the statistician in regulatory interactions in general and in Advisory Committee (AC) meetings, specifically.

Sponsor statisticians can add strong strategic value in preparation for and direct participation in meetings with regulators. Company statisticians are always part of the preparation for external regulatory interaction. Consequently, the opportunity is there to be more influential than their traditional role as a technical expert. The statistician should seize the opportunity to think strategically as well as technically to contribute more generally than just playing a purely statistical role. An example of strategic thinking might be to recommend that the company concentrate their position on selected studies that address the issue at hand more directly than other studies. This selection, of course, would not be based on which studies have favorable results, but could possibly be based on design features that make the study able to address the issue at hand. These distinctions are often subtle, but the statistician may be the best person to recognize them.

More generally, the statistician should insert him/herself into forming and developing the logic of the company's position. The strength of the company's position rests on the robustness of the study results, on the data. Consequently, the statistician should assess the strengths and weaknesses of the position. Knowledge of study results may not be sufficient to do this. Rather one must be thoroughly versed in all aspects of the issues at hand. The strategic statistician should anticipate and formulate responses to regulators' criticisms of study design, analytical methods, and strength of results. Armed with this preparation, the company statistician should not hesitate to jump into the discussion during the regulatory meeting. These meetings are almost always non-confrontational and quite cordial with both the regulators and sponsor looking for resolutions. In this spirit the sponsor statistician should look to be proactive and a strong participant to achieve the meeting goals. Simply providing a clarifying role and waiting to be invited into the discussion is not adequate statistical representation of the sponsor.

One of the more visible and important FDA interactions for the sponsor is an FDA Advisory Committee meeting. Advisory Committees consist of outside experts independent from FDA. These committees are convened by FDA to provide guidance and recommendations to FDA regarding the topic at hand. The topic is typically on a sponsor's application to market a new drug or on an important safety issue that has emerged post-approval for a specific drug or a class of drugs. FDA seeks guidance from the committee in the form of committee discussion and answers to specific questions posed by FDA. The sponsor is invited by FDA to present the data and any relevant information to the AC from the sponsor's perspective. Other regulatory bodies, such as EMA, have similar guidance mechanisms. Although our discussion of the statistician's role will be in the context of FDA Advisory Committee meetings, it is applicable to other regulatory settings.

The company statistician should have a prominent role in preparing for and participating in an FDA Advisory Committee meeting. The primary activities by the sponsor in preparation for an AC meeting is the preparation of the sponsor's Briefing Document (BD), the sponsor's presentation at the meeting, and responses to potential questions by the committee. The sponsor's BD contains all the data and information from the sponsor's perspective. The BD is submitted to FDA who then distributes it to the AC. Some recommendations for strategic statistical behavior in preparation for an AC meeting are.

- The statistician should strongly influence the presentation of the statistical results in the BD.
- The statistician should participate in formulating the sponsor's message and to assure that everyone is clear on the message to be delivered by the sponsor regarding statistical results/data.
- The statistician should study the BD and develop a framework to interpret its strengths and weaknesses. The statistician should be the internal expert on the company's briefing document.
- The statistician should endeavor to interact with and influence the leadership of the team rather than just defending top-down positions that may not be optimal.
- When outside experts are engaged by the company, the statistician should be proactive in briefing them on the critical issues and results.
- In preparatory meetings the statistician should bring up perceived weaknesses in the company's position, be it due to statistical methods/results or from a more general perspective. If the sponsor recognizes weaknesses and realizes that the statistician can articulate responses, then the role of the statistician at the AC meeting will be more prominent.

Sponsors often utilize mock AC meetings to prepare for the actual AC meeting. Internal and external experts form the mock panel, which is conducted in a manner similar to the real AC meeting. The sponsor makes its draft presentation and the panel asks questions to which the sponsor practices responses and the ability to call-up slides in support of the responses. This is often followed by a session where the internal and external panel members critique the presentation and responses to questions in order to make the sponsor aware of weaknesses and to strengthen the sponsor's position. This activity leads to an additional set of recommendations for strategic statistical behavior in preparation for an AC meeting.

- The statistician should develop his/her own set of statistical questions (e.g., weaknesses in statistical methods or ambiguity of results). The statistician should have answers to these statistical questions and practice delivering them clearly and succinctly.
- The statistician should realize that most questions have a statistical component to some extent and prepare answers for the statistical component in the context of the question.
- The statistician should take the initiative to conduct any additional analyses that may be needed at the actual AC or for the statistician's own additional understanding.
- The statistician should influence the development of answers to questions that are more in the clinical or regulatory domains. As recommended above, a framework to interpret the strengths and weaknesses of the BD will be helpful.
- The statistician should be assertive at the mock by being the person to answer questions related to statistics.
- In the post-mock critique session, the statistician should have their own recommendations for improvement and the rationale, and clarify important misperceptions by committee members or in sponsor answers. Often, the statistician is aware of weaknesses that others are not.

A strong role by the statistician during preparation should lead to a stronger formal presentation by the sponsor and stronger responses to potential committee questions to the sponsor.

At the actual AC meeting, the sponsor's statistician may make a formal presentation if statistical issues have been identified. If so, the statistician should be prepared to address clarifying and challenging questions on the presentation. Even in the absence of a formal presentation, most ACs will have at least one question that the statistician is the appropriate person to answer. If the proper up-front work has been done, the statistician should be identified as the person to respond. The sponsor statistician should be mindful that an AC statistician and an FDA statistician will also be present at the meeting. Often the FDA statistician will present his/her assessment of the sponsor's statistical methods and conclusions and may also present alternative analyses. The statistician on the AC is usually an academic statistician with expertise in clinical-trial methods. The AC statistician does not make a formal presentation but often takes a strong role in AC discussions. This leads to a final set of recommendations for the statistician at the actual AC.

- Sponsors spend a great deal of time preparing answers to potential questions at the AC. However, the actual questions are almost never the precise questions that were anticipated and prepared for. Therefore, instead of using a prepared answer, it is important to understand the question from the perspective of the AC member. It is advisable to use the framework of issues derived from the BD to answer the question in an informational manner, emphasizing strengths but not overlooking weaknesses.
- Related to point 1, the statistician should answer the question that is being asked in a succinct and precise manner, without offering answers to questions that are not asked or speculating. However, the statistician should not hesitate to put his/her answer in a broader positive context.
- If the question is related to differences between the sponsor and FDA analytical methods, it is prudent to try to show that the analyses are complimentary rather than in conflict, particularly if there are no substantive differences in conclusions.
- The statistician should refrain from statistical jargon, even if addressing a question from the AC statistician, since the intended audience is the entire AC committee. The statistician should put the question and the answer in terms readily understandable by all committee members. In particular, the statistician's demeanor should never be contentious, but informative and collaborative.
- Most questions at an AC meeting have a statistical component, but the statistician is not the primary responder for the sponsor. These questions can sometimes turn into a statistical discussion. The statistician should

not hesitate to attempt to clarify the discussion. The proper way to do this is by alerting the main sponsor representative who will then ask the AC chair if the sponsor statistician can address the committee.

- The statistician must remember that there is a protocol that governs AC meetings regarding who can speak and when. The set of questions addressed to the sponsor directly after the sponsor presentation is the primary time, if not the only time, that the sponsor can make points to the committee. Consequently, any important statistical points that the sponsor wants to make must be made during this time.

Three actual examples are described briefly to illustrate some behaviors recommended in this section.

Example 1. This AC meeting addressed whether a large, long-term randomized study looking at cardiovascular events should be stopped. Since the time the study began, additional information from an indirect meta-analysis of randomized studies along with studies from observational databases seemed to indicate that one study drug was safer than the two other drugs in the study and thus the study should be stopped. In preparation for the AC meeting the sponsor statistician made the point that the meta-analysis did not support the safety of one drug due to the indirect nature of the comparisons, and that the results of observational studies were not supportive of stopping the ongoing study. As a result, the statistician made a formal presentation at the AC meeting that equipoise remains among the three study drugs and that the study should not be stopped. This led to an active interaction between the sponsor statistician and the AC and with the AC voting to continue the study. The large randomized study was continued to completion and the final analysis did not support the results of the meta-analysis or the observational studies.

Example 2. This AC meeting addressed the association of serious neuropsychiatric events with treatment for smoking cessation. A large randomized trial of three active treatments and placebo was conducted. The focus of the AC meeting was on a particular treatment of smoking cessation. The sponsor's conclusion was that there was no association between the neuropsychiatric events and the sponsor's treatment. Prior to the meeting the sponsor received the FDA briefing document that indicated that the FDA statistician conducted an analysis using different methods than the sponsor that might cast doubt on the sponsor's conclusion. The sponsor statistician recognized that this difference in methods could lead to a discussion at the AC meeting and constructed a rationale showing that the analyses were not in conflict but were complementary. In addition, the statistician anticipated that, if not the treatment, it would be effective to identify the determinants of these events in patients attempting to quit smoking and to show they are the same for placebo and active-treatment patients. At the AC meeting, the statistician made both presentations that were helpful in an AC vote in the sponsor's favor.

Example 3. This AC meeting addressed the approval of a treatment for Post-Traumatic Stress Disorder (PTSD). The sponsor's studies showed that the treatment was efficacious in women with PTSD, but not men. Although there were two positive studies overall and the treatment-by-sex differential was a secondary finding, the sponsor statistician anticipated that this treatment-by-sex interaction could become an AC meeting issue. The statistician, as due diligence, conducted many additional analyses exploring possible reasons for this interaction. No strong reason was found but there was some evidence of efficacy in men for whom sexual abuse was the predominantly precipitating traumatic event. The statistician was called upon at the AC meeting to present many of these exploratory analyses. The treatment was approved without a labeling restriction to women.

3.5 STATISTICAL ROLE IN PROMOTIONAL MATERIAL AND MEDICAL COMMUNICATION

An important activity for both the pharmaceutical company and the regulators is product promotion and medical communication. This activity is highly regulated and highly scrutinized. If not done properly there can be major consequences to public health and to the reputation of the company, as well as financial penalties. On the otherhand, clinical trials contain much information outside of the primary endpoint and it is helpful to prescribers, payers, and patients to communicate this information. This point of view has been recognized by FDA in their 2018 guidance, "Medical product communications that are consistent with the FDA-required labeling." This guidance reduces the degree of support for a promotional piece from "substantial evidence" to "sufficient evidence" that is "scientifically appropriate and statistically sound." However, the material will be judged as not acceptable if it leaves a misleading impression. The need for statistical input in this area is self-evident. The following are general statistical points that should be considered on review of promotional material in order to assess whether the material could be considered misleading.

- The treatment effect or information that is promoted should be derived from all studies that address the research question, i.e., it is not seen in a single study if more than one study addresses the issue – inclusive, not selective of positive findings. Of course, there may only be one study that addresses the issue in which case it should be statistically strong.
- The effect among the studies should be consistent, i.e., heterogeneity of effect is small. One should consider whether the material is consistent with the totality of the sponsor's data.
- To address the potential for the criticism of *post hoc* analyses, in the case of multiple secondary endpoints, there should be an appropriate multiplicity procedure to control the overall Type I error, which is a major regulatory concern.
- If there is no multiplicity issue for a particular finding, then the clinical importance of the finding and any prior justification or information to support the finding would support the promotional material. In this regard, the results are clinically important (informative to prescriber, patient, payer) and hence statistically stronger (viewed as less *post hoc*) if the analyses address, for example, aspects of the primary endpoint, components of a composite primary endpoint, dependence of response on disease severity, onset/duration of effect, or the treatment effect in clinically important subgroups. Although FDA has frowned on the promotion of subgroup effects in the past, the current guidance specifically allows for subgroup results under certain circumstances. This is consistent with the development of targeted therapy, for example, in oncology, where the results in tumors with or without a genetic marker would be important.
- In reviewing promotional material, the statistician should be cognizant of the clinical context and prior justification for the material, so it is not criticized as data mining.

In the guidance, for promotional material to be not misleading, FDA stresses that product communications should not overstate the findings or the conclusions that can be drawn from such studies or analyses. The presentation requires proper contextual language including limitations of the strength of evidence (FDA 2018). This is where statistical input is critical to get the context correct.

3.6 CONCLUDING REMARKS

The main purpose of this chapter is to describe behaviors that can lead to a strong strategic role for the statistician internally and in regulatory and other external interactions. The statistician should establish a strategic and influential role internally so that there is a natural inclusion of the statistician as a strategic player in regulatory interaction. While the recommendations given in this chapter are intended to have general application, the statistician should interpret them in the context of the specific regulatory setting. As indicated in the introduction, the importance of statistics and statisticians has been firmly established in the pharmaceutical industry. It will benefit the drug-development process to extend that importance into the regulatory sphere.

BIBLIOGRAPHY

DeMets, D., Furberg, C., Friedman, L. (2006) *Data Monitoring in Clinical Trials: A Case Studies Approach.* New York: Springer.

Ellenberg, S., Fleming, T., DeMets, D. (2002) *Data Monitoring Committees in Clinical Trials: A Practical Perspective.* Hoboken, New Jersey: John Wiley & Sons.

Emir, B., Amaratunga, D., Beltangady, M. et al. (2013) Generating productive dialogue between consulting statisticians and their clients in the pharmaceutical and medical research settings. Open Access. Medical Statistics . 3: 51–56.

European Medicines Agency (2005) Guideline on data monitoring committees. www.ema.europa.eu/en/documents/scientific-guideline/guideline-data-monitoring-committees_en.pdf.

Food and Drug Administration (2006) Guidance for clinical trial sponsors. Establishment and operation of clinical trial data monitoring committees. www.fda.gov/media/75398/download.

Food and Drug Administration (2018) Guidance documents/Medical product communications are consistent FDA-required labeling questions and answers. www.fda.gov/regulatory-information/search-fda-guidance-documents/medical-product-communications-are-consistent-fda-required-labeling-questions-and-answers.

Grieve, A. P. (2002) Do statisticians count? A personal view. *Pharmaceutical Statistics*. 1(1): 35–43.

Grieve, A. P. (2005) The professionalization of the "shoe clerk". *Journal of the Royal Statistical Society Series A (Statistics in Society)*. 168(4): 639–656.

Herson, J. (2009) *Data and Safety Monitoring Committees in Clinical Trials*. New York: Chapman & Hall/CRC.

Lewi, P. J. (2005) The role of statistics in the success of a pharmaceutical research laboratory: A historical case description. *Journal of Chemometrics*. 19: 282–287.

Marquardt, D. W. (1987) The importance of statisticians. *Journal of American Statistical Association*. 82(397): 1–7.

Rockhold, F. W. (2009) Strategic use of statistical thinking in drug development. *Statistics in Medicine*. 19: 3211–3217.

Unwin A. (2007) Statistical consulting interactions: A personal view. *Advances in Statistical Analysis*. 91(4): 349–359.

CHAPTER 4

Emerging Topics

4.1 THE USE OF RWE TO SUPPORT LICENSING AND LABEL ENHANCEMENT

4.1.1 Introduction

Regulatory agencies rely mostly on data from randomized controlled trials (RCTs) to make major decision relating to the safety and efficacy of alternative treatment options. As pointed out in earlier sections, this is in part due to the internal validity of RCTs, relative to non-randomized studies. However, there are situations where RCTs may not be appropriate for operational or ethical reasons. Under such circumstances, it may be necessary to use information from observational studies.

Real-world data (RWD) has been defined as "data relating to patient health status and/or the delivery of health care routinely collected from a variety of sources," while real-world evidence (RWE) pertains to the "evidence about the usage and potential benefits or risks of a medical product derived from analysis of RWD" (US FDA 2019b). Historically, RWE from observational studies has been typically used by regulators for post-approval safety monitoring and regulatory decisions. Healthcare providers employ RWE in the assessment of benefits and risks from pharmacoeconomic perspectives in order to support coverage decisions and guidelines for use in clinical practice. More recently, pharmaceutical companies have been using RWD to generate RWE to support additional efficacy or safety labeling for the therapeutic product label. Thus, with progress in health information technology and modern analytics, RWE can now be used to address important regulatory questions and to demonstrate the value of medical products. As a result, regulatory agencies have begun formulating programs to promote the application of RWE. A case in point is the *21st Century Cures Act of 2016* intended to establish a framework for use of RWE in regulatory decision-making in the US (Public Law No: 114–255 (December 13, 2016)). In addition, FDA has issued important guidance on the topic of RWD and RWE (see, e.g., FDA 2018b and FDA 2018c)

On the other hand, there are many limitations of observational studies, especially in the context of regulatory use. Although randomization can be employed in real-world settings (Sherman et al. 2016), observational studies are non-interventional and hence randomization is absent. One inherent major problem of nonrandom assignment of subjects to treatment is the likely bias in the assessment of treatment comparisons. Biases arise from the lack of comparability among treatment groups with respect to known and unknown confounding factors (Deeks et al. 2003). Other shortcomings include data quality, accessibility of data sources, and the protection of privacy and confidentiality of patients (Alemayehu and Mardekian 2011). Recent studies also suggest that results of observational studies tend to depend on trial design, data source, and analytical procedures (Madigan et al. 2013a). This goes to the heart of the generalizability of results of observational studies. Bartlett et al. (2019) presented research results on the feasibility of RWD to replicate RCTs using US-based clinical trials published in high-impact journals in 2017. Their study, which had certain limitations, reported that only 15% of the clinical trials could be replicated using currently available RWD.

As a result, there has been a growing body of literature on approaches to maximize the value of real-world evidence (RWE) in healthcare decision-making, both from the methodological as well as the operational perspectives (Berger et al. 2014; Rosenbaum and Rubin 1983; Waning and Montagne 2001). Unsurprisingly, regulatory agencies are also in the process of evaluating the potential of RWE in drug development and approval (FDA 2018c; Sutter 2016).

In this chapter, we summarize some of the statistical and regulatory issues with the use of RWE in drug development, with particular reference to recent developments in the US and other regions. A brief outline is provided regarding the common approaches used in the design analysis and reporting of observational studies. In addition, selected examples are provided to highlight the current regulatory viewpoints pertaining to the role of RWE in drug development.

4.1.2 Methodological and Operational Considerations

In the literature, a confounder is defined as a variable that is associated both with the response and the treatments under study. In RCTs, randomization ensures comparability of treatment groups with respect to observed as well as latent confounders (Collins and Lanza 2009). In the absence of randomization, it is generally impossible to eliminate the impacts of all potential confounders. In some cases, such as confounding by indication, which is common in drug safety studies where the indication is also a risk factor for the outcome, the associated bias cannot be completely removed by design or modeling, when no control exists for the underlying condition (Bosco et al. 2010; Psaty and Siscovick 2010). Therefore, best practices should be used in the design and analysis of data from observational studies, and caution should be exercised in the interpretation of the accompanying results.

Alternative design options are available for observational studies. Prospective cohort studies are often used to compare treatment regimens based on subjects that use the drug of interest and others that use a suitably chosen comparator, both prospectively identified with respect to predefined criteria. The subjects are then followed over time and the outcome of interest compared in the two groups, using models that adjust for relevant confounders. Such designs tend to be resource-intensive and generally require lengthy time for data collection, particularly for rare events. In some cases, retrospective cohort studies, which are relatively less costly, may be executed; however, such studies may be limited by the availability of data for analysis (Kleinbaum et al. 2013).

Matched case-control designs often prove to be appealing since they are cheaper and less time-consuming than prospective cohort studies. In such designs, subjects having a given outcome (cases) are matched to those without the outcome (controls) according to a prespecified matching criterion. The rates of exposures in the two groups are then compared using analysis methods that take into account the potential correlation introduced by the matching. The selection of a suitable control group is essential to obtaining valid results. Case-control studies tend to suffer from selection bias, and lack of generalizability of the results, since study subjects are selected according to the outcome values (Kleinbaum et al. 2013; Madigan et al. 2013b).

A common approach for handling observed confounders is the use of traditional models, such as the standard linear model, generalized linear models, or a Cox proportional hazards model, in which the confounders are included as covariates. While these procedures have many desirable properties, including ease of interpretation, they can be sensitive to departure from model assumptions. For example, they may lead to misleading results in the presence of multicollinearity or influential points. They may also lead to inefficient estimators when the number of covariates is large relative to the number of observations. Recent approaches that involve regularization, including ridge regression and the lasso (Tibshirani 1996) have been proposed as viable solutions to mitigate some of the issues (see, e.g., Hastie et al. 2009). However, the results based on regression approaches cannot be fully relied upon to address confounding issues.

The propensity-score technique, introduced in Rosenbaum and Rubin (1983), is one of the most widely used methods for handling observed confounders. The underlying principle is based on the concept of counterfactual causality (Heckman 2005). More specifically, given two treatment groups, denoted by Z, having a value of 1 if the subject is exposed, and 0 otherwise, the propensity score (PS) for an individual is defined as the conditional probability of being treated given the covariates:

$$p_i = Pr(Z = 1 | \text{ covariates for subject } i).$$

The propensity scores are typically estimated using standard logistic-regression models. The estimated individual subject propensity scores can then be used in 1:1 or M:1 matching, grouping subjects with respect to their PS values (D'Agostino 1998). A drawback of matching is a potential loss of observations if there are not suitable matches at the low or high end of the PS. The observations are then trimmed, and the remaining matched subjects are analyzed. As in the case of matching by individual characteristics, the PS matching will introduce correlation into the matched observations that should be taken into account in the analysis.

Alternative approaches are available to perform analyses involving PS matching. In some applications, the estimated propensity score is included as one of the covariates in the model. However, this approach has been shown to give biased estimates (Austin 2009a; Imbens 2004). Another approach concerns stratification, in which subjects are categorized into disjoint subsets based on prespecified PS thresholds. A method proposed by Cochran (1968) consists in dividing subjects into five equal-size groups. In this framework, the analysis may be performed by pooling stratum-specific estimates by weighing the stratum-specific estimates by the inverse of their variances or using standard techniques, such as analysis of variance (ANOVA), logistic regression, or Cox proportional hazards models, with the PS strata included as a stratification term in the model. If each treatment group is not adequately represented in each stratum, the method may suffer from loss of information. Stratifying by PS groups has also been shown to be a good diagnostic method to assess effect modification as well as residual confounding and to elucidate the treatment effect with respect to the original confounding variables (Gaffney and Mardekian, 2009).

A method that involves assigning each subject a weight equal to the inverse of the probability of receiving the treatment the subject actually received is the so-called *inverse probability of treatment weighting* (IPTW). In the abovementioned notation, the weight for individual i is given by:

$$w_i = \frac{Z_i}{p_i} + \frac{(1-Z_i)}{(1-p_i)}$$

Given outcome Y, the average treatment effect δ is estimated by:

$$\hat{\delta} = \frac{1}{n}\sum_{i=1}^{n}\frac{Z_iY_i}{p_i} - \frac{1}{n}\sum_{i=1}^{n}\frac{(1-Z_i)Y_i}{1-p_i}$$

Inference about δ may be performed using suitable estimates of the standard error of $\hat{\delta}$ (Lunceford and Davidian 2004). One limitation of the IPTW approach is that weights may be unstable for subjects with small values of the PS (Robins et al. 2000). The rationale for the IPTW analysis is that subjects with a relatively high p_i are overrepresented in the treatment group and thus their observations are down weighted while the reverse is true for the control subjects.

The pros and cons of the abovementioned procedures may be found in Austin (2007; 2009b). It is noted that in certain settings PS matching may not be always preferable compared with conventional multivariable methods (Sturmer et al. 2006), and that the performance of the method is in general dependent on the appropriateness of the variables included in the construction of the scores. Further, in the face of high dimensionality and collinearity, the models may not perform adequately (Schneeweiss et al. 2009). For a discussion of use of modern analytic approaches, see, e.g., Setoguchi et al. (2008).

Instrumental variable (IV) techniques are often used to handle unmeasured confounders in observational studies (Newhouse and McClellan 1998). An unmeasured confounder may simply be a confounder such as disease severity at the time of treatment initiation, which is not captured in the RWD or, more subtly, it may be the reasons why the prescriber decides to select one treatment over the alternative for a given subject. That is, clinical judgment often leads to confounding that cannot be controlled for by any measured subject characteristics. To be implemented reliably, an IV must satisfy two conditions: (1) it must be strongly associated with treatment; and 2) it does not have a direct effect on the outcome variable, but only through the treatment variable. An example of an IV construction may be interruptions in medical practice, which may be a consequence of an important innovation. Another involves treatment preference, independent of patient factors. Instances of the latter may include distance to specialists (McClellan et al. 1994); geographic areas (Stukel et al. 2007); physician prescribing preference (Brookhart et al. 2006); and hospital formulary (Schneeweiss et al. 2007). The IV is included in the analysis as a covariate or stratification variable to adjust for unmeasured confounders. However, one can never be certain that unmeasured confounding has been adequately addressed and it remains a limitation to the analysis of observational data. An alternative method to address unmeasured confounding is by a tipping point analysis. In this approach the amount of unmeasured confounding that would be required to change the study conclusion is estimated.

In addition to the methodological issues discussed above, effective use of data from observational studies requires addressing important operational challenges. Since healthcare data may come from different sources, including electronic health records (EHRs) and claims databases, they typically require special provisions for data storage, computing environment, data standards, and protection of privacy and confidentiality (Alemayehu and Mardekian 2011). Depending on the sources, different nomenclatures, coding conventions, and units are often used for medical terms. Since data collection is not performed for the purpose of research, data entry errors are common, often leading to such issues as miss-classification, missing values, and outliers. In addition, most of the available data may be unstructured.

As a result, concerted efforts are required by various stakeholders to establish a framework for the harmonization of healthcare data. Recent activities in this regard include increased use of the *International Classification of Diseases, Ninth Revision, Clinical Modification* (ICD-9-CM) to code and classify diagnoses from inpatient and outpatient records. The National Drug Code (NDC) scheme, which is maintained by the US Food and Drug Administration (FDA), is another tool for coding prescription drugs and insulin products. In addition, some initiatives are underway in the US to harmonize data collection across states (Porter et al. 2015).

4.1.3 Current Regulatory Landscape

Despite the growing attention given to the potential use of data from observational studies in evidence-based medicine, the regulatory requirement is still an evolving concept. Some of the important guidelines relating to the design, analysis, and reporting of observational studies have been issued by professional societies and other stakeholders. Notable examples include, the recommendations of the International Society for Pharmacoeconomics and Outcomes Research (ISPOR) (Berger et al. 2009); the STrengthening the Reporting of OBservational studies in Epidemiology (STROBE) statement (von Elm et al. 2008); and other resources for evaluating nonrandomized studies of comparative effectiveness (Deeks et al. 2003).

In the US, following the promulgation of the *21st Century Cures Act of 2016*, the FDA has issued a framework for the use of RWE in regulatory decision-making (FDA 2018b). Key aspects of the framework include developing guidelines relating to: a) Whether the RWD are fit for use; b) Whether the trial or study design used to generate RWE can provide adequate scientific evidence to answer or help answer the regulatory question; and c) Whether the study conduct meets FDA regulatory requirements (e.g., for study monitoring and data collection).

With respect to effectiveness objectives, regulators are reluctant to draw a causal inference when treatment assignment is due to physician judgment, rather than randomly. FDA has stated that this must be addressed to support the acceptability of observational studies for effectiveness decisions (FDA 2018b, 2018c). There are examples of concordance between randomized trials and observational studies reaching similar conclusions about treatment effect (Anglemyer et al. 2014; Benson and Hartz 2000); however, there are also examples of discordant results (Cooper et al. 2014; Guadino et al. 2018; Hemkens et al. 2016). There have been recent efforts to use rigorous design and statistical methods to replicate randomized trial results with observational studies and to develop general rules to strengthen the validity of results in observational study designs (Franklin and Schneeweiss 2017). However, because of the discordant results given above and the uncertainty of the validity of observational results, it is unlikely that regulators will rely on results from observational studies for the purpose of effectiveness, except in certain special situations.

One important area of interest relates to enhancing non-randomized, single-arm trials through the use of external controls. Although the external control arm could use data from past RCTs, suitably chosen RWD might also be used to construct external controls. However, as highlighted elsewhere in this monograph, external controls have their own limitations, including lack of comparability of patient populations, lack of standardized diagnostic criteria, dissimilarity of outcome measures, and variability in follow-up procedures. The FDA Framework is anticipated to provide further guidance on the use of RWD to generate external control arms, complementing the ICH E10 guideline (ICH 2000).

Earlier, the US FDA issued a guidance document pertaining to the use of RWE to support regulatory decision-making for medical devices (FDA 2001). The document addresses important issues that arise in the evaluation of real-world data, including methodological rigor and data quality. More recently, a related guidance was issued, including recommendations for evaluating data sources used in pharmacoepidemiologic safety studies (FDA 2013).

There is a growing interest in pragmatic clinical trials, which involve randomization, and are typically integrated into routine clinical care. The study protocols for such trials specify minimal inclusion and exclusion criteria, and no treatment requirement other than the randomized assignment to one of the groups. Such trials may use EHRs or claims data to capture primary and secondary endpoints (see, e.g., Hernandez et al. 2015) or may be registry-based (e.g., Fröbert et al. 2013).

Incidentally, there are several examples of RWE use in regulatory settings, including label expansion for new indications, fulfilling postapproval commitments, and even initial approval based upon external controls, especially in areas of high unmet medical need (Baumfeld Andre et al. 2019). Some use cases relate to label expansion based on EHRs, or postmarketing reports of claims databases. A recent example is the approval of palbociclib

(Ibrance) for the treatment of male breast cancer, expanding the earlier indication for the treatment of HR+, HER2- advanced/metastatic breast cancer in females (FDA 2019a). The approval was based on post-marketing reports and EHRs as part of the totality of evidence. Real-world data from EHRs showed encouraging signals of response rates with Ibrance, a CDK4/6 inhibitor in combination with an aromatase inhibitor or fulvestrant in the male patient population. The data also suggest that the safety of Ibrance in male patients was consistent with the tolerability observed in female patients who received palbociclib.

An example of label expansion using a pragmatic study concerns paliperidone palmitate, originally indicated for the treatment of schizophrenia in adults and treatment of schizoaffective disorder in adults as monotherapy and as an adjunct to mood stabilizers or antidepressants (Alphs et al. 2016).

Approvals have also been granted based on historical controls. An example is the accelerated approval of eteplirsen for Duchenne muscular dystrophy. The approval of eteplirsen used data on a historic control arm from a registry database (Mendell et al. 2016). In another case, label expansion was granted for blinatumomab based on the results of a single-arm trial supported by RWE to include indication for patients with minimal residual disease in which cancer cells are present at a low level that cannot be detected microscopically (Gokbuget et al. 2018).

4.1.4 Concluding Remarks

In this chapter, we considered some of the issues associated with the use of RWE in regulatory settings, and highlighted steps that need to be taken to maximize the evidentiary value of such data in drug development. Although the traditional RCT paradigm is the default approach for regulatory decision-making, there are considerable opportunities for RWE in label expansion and even initial approvals. With the growing cost of conducting RCTs, and the infeasibility of generating the requisite evidence for rare diseases, observational studies and RWD have garnered increased attention to support regulatory decision-making.

Historically, RWE from observational studies has been routinely accepted for satisfying postapproval safety commitments. With the development of guidelines and best practices, and gradual evolution of regulatory opinions, examples now abound illustrating regulatory decision-making based on RWE. Hybrid designs that incorporate randomization and minimal protocol requirements can be used to generate regulatory-grade evidence, especially in areas of unmet medical needs. In other cases, external controls involving RWD can be used to buttress single-arm trials.

Despite the various examples of approvals using RWE, the regulatory landscape pertaining to such data is by and large an evolving process. The onus is first on the sponsor to assess the appropriateness of the use of RWD from an observational database for the sponsor's specific research purpose and that the results will have scientific rigor. There are myriad medical, statistical, regulatory issues to consider, as well as the nature of the observational database itself. An observational study should never be conducted simply because it may be more expedient than a clinical trial. Therefore, it is essential for sponsors to engage regulatory authorities early and obtain alignment of expectations. To facilitate the discussion with regulators and maximize the possibility of positive outcome, sponsors should apply best practices for study design, methodological rigor, and data quality. Special attention should also be paid to regulatory requirements for record retention, auditing, patient privacy, clinical endpoint validity, and reporting of study results. Sponsors should also put in place standard operating procedures to ensure transparency, including prespecification of protocols and analysis methods, data-quality assurance, and registration of studies and study results.

4.2 PATIENT-REPORTED OUTCOMES IN REGULATORY SETTINGS

4.2.1 Introduction

According to a recent guidance document issued by the US FDA, patient-reported outcomes (PROs) are defined as "any report of the status of a patient's health condition that comes directly from the patient, without interpretation of the patient's response by a clinician or anyone else" (FDA 2009). Thus, PROs may include a range of such subjective outcomes as symptoms (e.g., pain, fatigue, nausea, or vomiting), functioning (physical, emotional, or social), health-related quality of life (HRQOL), or preference about a given treatment (Drummond et al. 2005). PRO data is captured directly from the patients using a suitable instrument, which consists of a questionnaire and accompanying instruction and documentation in support of its use. While a PRO is typically measured by self-report, in some situations it may be captured by interview, in which case the interviewer is expected to record only the patient's response. It is noted that certain symptoms or other concepts that are known only to the patient (e.g., pain severity) can only be measured using PRO instruments.

Pharmaceutical companies and regulatory agencies pay due attention to the collection, analysis, and reporting of PROs (see, e.g., Alemayehu and Cappelleri 2012; 2014). The importance of PROs stems from the fact that there is a growing focus on patient-centric healthcare system. The US FDA acknowledges that evidence from a well-defined and reliable PRO instrument collected through an appropriately designed investigation can be used to support a claim in medical product labeling (FDA 2009). In the European Union (EU), the EMA has recognized the fact that the "experience of patients of how a treatment impacts on their well-being and everyday life is an important aspect of the evaluation of the clinical benefits of new medicines" (EMA 2016). In addition, PROs can be used as evidence to support health-technology assessment (HTA) decisions and payer negotiations (Zagadailov 2013). PROs are, therefore, routinely included as an integral component of most drug-development plans, often starting in early-phase trial designs (Basch 2016).

Since PROs are subjective in nature, their acceptance as a basis for the assessment of the relative benefits and risks of alternative treatment options is dependent on the validity and reliability of the instruments used to generate the data. In addition, it is essential to ensure that PROs are developed following standardized approaches, so that results can be compared or synthesized across measures, and that the burden on patients is reduced to a minimum. The Patient-Reported Outcome Measurement Information System, or PROMIS (Cella 2007), which was launched in 2005 through a National Institutes of Health (NIH) Roadmap Initiative, is an example of ongoing efforts intended to enhance the development, use, and interpretation of PROs (see, e.g., DeWalt 2007).

In the following, we provide a high-level summary of pertinent aspects of PRO-instrument development as well as data collection, analysis, and reporting, with emphasis on the issues that are germane to their effective use in clinical trials and regulatory submissions. For a more in-depth discussion of these issues, the reader is referred to Cappelleri et al. (2013).

4.2.2 Development and Validation of PRO Instruments

The development of a PRO instrument that is intended to be used to generate evidence for regulatory or other healthcare decision-making requires a rigorous evaluation process, involving both qualitative and quantitative methods. The initial step often comprises a thorough review of the available literature to confirm the need for a new instrument and to understand the nature of the measures that are already in use for related purposes. The next step would be development and assessment of a conceptual framework that guarantees that the issues of most relevance to the patient are captured. The concept of interest may involve a single item (e.g., pain intensity), or require multiple items (e.g., physical function). In the case of the latter, it is critical to establish how individual items are associated with each other and each domain, and how domains are associated with each other and the general concept of interest. Figure 4.1 adapted from FDA (2009), illustrates the interrelationships of items and domains in a conceptual framework of a PRO instrument.

Once the conceptual framework is confirmed, other properties of the instrument will need to be established, including content validity, reliability, construct validity, and ability to detect change.

The assessment of content validity, which requires evidence that the instrument measures the concept of interest, includes analyzing data collected from focus groups (Patrick et al. 2011a; 2011b). Content validity depends on a number of factors, including whether item generation includes input from the target patient population; appropriateness of the recall period for the instrument; the mode of administration (i.e., whether self-administration, interview, or both); relevance of the response options (e.g., visual analog scale, Likert scale, etc.); scoring of items and domains; and respondent burden.

Construct validity involves establishing whether observed relationships between measures gathered using the instrument and results gathered

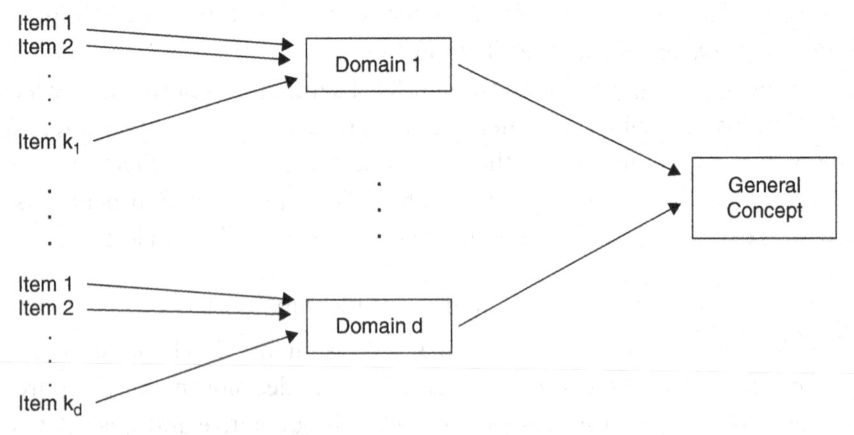

FIGURE 4.1 Illustration of a Conceptual Framework of a PRO Instrument

using other measures are in congruence with preexisting hypotheses about those relationships (i.e., discriminant and convergent validity), as well as whether the instrument can differentiate between clinically distinct groups (i.e., known groups validity). In addition, an instrument's floor/ceiling effects are assessed to determine the appropriate use of the instrument for a given condition. The ability of the instrument to discriminate among patients is characterized by assessing the variability in responses when the instrument is administered. Further, an instrument's ability to capture responsiveness to meaningful change may be determined by comparing the change in PRO scores against the change in other similar measures or a gold standard (criterion validity).

The assessment of the reliability of an instrument consists in evaluation of its ability to yield consistent, reproducible results. This may include determination of reproducibility (e.g., test-retest reliability), internal consistency (e.g., agreement among the observed responses to different questions), as well as inter-interviewer reproducibility, if applicable. Internal consistency is assessed with respect to item-to-item correlations (often using Cronbach's alpha), whereas test-retest reliability may be assessed based on an analysis of variance involving repeated measurements on the same set of subjects.

4.2.3 Statistical Considerations

From a statistical perspective, the analysis and reporting of PRO data require tackling considerable challenges, including handling of missing values and multiplicity of endpoints, as well as determination of interpretable response criteria.

In PRO data, missingness may occur in a variety of ways. As in other clinical endpoints, the data may be missing for an entire visit due to loss to follow up or other reasons. In other cases, data may be missing for certain components of a multi-item instrument (item-level missing). In the latter situation, some instruments may have accompanying documentations for handling the missing items (Cappelleri et al. 2013). In general, alternative strategies may be employed to impute the missing values, under various assumptions about the mechanism that generated the missingness. A common approach is to use single-imputation methods for missing item-level data (Fairclough 2010). However, even when the assumptions about the missing-data mechanism are satisfied, such techniques tend to underestimate the variability of the estimators of interest, thereby invalidating the accompanying inferential results. When the assumption of missing at random (MAR) is satisfied, multiple-imputation techniques or, in the case of longitudinal data, mixed models for repeated measures (MMRM) may be used (see, e.g., Carpenter and Kenward 2013).

In practice, it may not be possible to verify the assumption of MAR. It is therefore critical to confirm the results under MAR using alternative sensitivity analyses corresponding to the same parameter of interest (Little and Rubin 2002). For longitudinal data, some of the commonly used approaches include pattern-mixture models (Little 1993) and selection models (Little and Rubin 2019). Selection models, which specify the joint distribution of the outcome and missing-data mechanism as a function of the marginal distribution of the measurements and the conditional distribution of the missing data given the measurements, are highly dependent on strong assumptions about the model and dropout patterns. In contrast, pattern-mixture models, which express the joint distribution in terms of the marginal distribution of the missing data and the conditional distribution of the measurements given missing data, tend to rely on classification of individuals based on time of dropout. A key limitation of the latter approach is under-identifiability, since some parameters cannot be directly estimated due to inadequate information.

An approach that is gaining popularity involves performing a series of analyses searching for a tipping point that reverses the study conclusion (see, e.g., O'Kelly and Ratitch 2014). The intended purpose of this approach is to assess the degree of departures from the missingness assumption that would overturn the findings obtained using MAR-based models.

Since there is no universally accepted approach to handle missing values at the analysis stage, it is highly recommended to minimize the occurrence of missing data by employing best practices at the design and conduct stages of the trial. To the extent possible, a minimally required number of instruments should be included in the study, and the frequency of data collection from the participants should be limited to the time points that are absolutely necessary to address the research hypothesis. Further, automated data collection tools, such as ePROs, should be used, if available. During the conduct phases, several proactive measures may be taken, including training investigators, implementing incentives to investigators and participants, and maintaining contact information of participants for potential follow-up.

As mentioned above, for longitudinal PRO data, suitable linear models may be implemented (see, e.g., Cappelleri et al. 2013; Fairclough 2010; Fitzmaurice et al. 2011; Hedeker and Gibbons 2006; Singer and Willett 2003). In addition, other nonstandard techniques may also be used, including item-response theory (IRT), discussed earlier (Cappelleri et al. 2013; de Ayala 2005; Hambleton et al. 1991; Hays et al. 2000).

Since PRO analyses typically involve multiple endpoints, appropriate methods should be prospectively specified and implemented to control the Type I error rate. If PROs are considered secondary endpoints, the additional endpoints may be tested sequentially following a significant test on the primary endpoint, each at the usual alpha = 0.05 level of statistical significance. In cases where the primary analysis concerns two or more primary endpoints, a suitable statistical procedure should be applied for multiplicity adjustment, including a gate-keeping strategy involving a hierarchy of comparisons that should first be satisfied before others are considered for testing. Other more conventional approaches that may be used when a restriction of the hierarchy is not feasible or practical include such conventional methods, as Bonferroni, the step-down or step-up tests, and prospective alpha allocations schemes. In certain situation, in which it is reasonable to combine individual items, composite endpoints may be employed to avoid multiplicity issues.

A commonly used psychometric approach for the assessment of validity involves the use of exploratory and confirmatory factor analyses. The former is used to generate hypotheses about the concepts represented by the various items, and to guide decisions about the items that are conceived to be of relevance. In confirmatory factor analysis, the goal is to establish the acceptability of a prespecified hypothesis about various aspects of the measure. Alternatively, IRT may also be used to assess validity. In this approach, the probability of response to an item is expressed as a function of certain latent attributes and parameters. Other ways of assessing validity, mentioned earlier, may include demonstration of correlations with existing measures that address the same concept (convergent validity), or that assess other concepts (divergent validity).

4.2.4 Regulatory Considerations

As pointed out earlier, the US FDA generally accepts evidence from a well-defined and reliable PRO instrument in appropriately designed trials to support a claim in medical product labeling. The role of a PRO endpoint (i.e., whether primary, key secondary, or exploratory) should be clearly prespecified in the trial protocol, including the statistical methods that would be used to analyze the data. Some of the characteristics of PRO instruments that are routinely reviewed by the US FDA include: instrument's measurement properties; the concepts being measured; number of items, medical condition, and population for intended use; data collection method; respondent burden; recall period; and translation or cultural adaptation availability, among others (FDA 2009).

Definition of an appropriate PRO endpoint may involve a fixed time point or a suitable summary statistic across time points. The defined endpoint is expected to reflect the objective of the given analysis and will determine the type of statistical procedure to be used. For example, an ordinal or continuous PRO score at a fixed time point in an RCT may be analyzed using standard parametric (e.g., two-sample t-test or analysis of variance) or nonparametric (e.g., Wilcoxon rank-sum test or Kruskal–Wallis test) analyses. In situations where it is desired to adjust for potential imbalances in baseline scores, alternative approaches may be employed, including computation of the change from baseline or the percentage change from baseline for each patient, with subsequent comparison between arms based on an analysis of covariance (ANCOVA). Similarly, binary PRO scores at a fixed time point may be analyzed using chi-squared or similar tests, or a logistic regression incorporating relevant covariates.

Suitably defined summary measures can serve several purposes, including facilitating interpretation, selecting analytical approaches, and reducing dimensions by combining data across scales and/or time points into a single score. However, the choice of the summary measures should be done judiciously, taking into account the impact of any missing values and the potential loss of information in the process of constructing the measures. Commonly used examples include, the average, maximum, minimum, or last observed postbaseline score; slope across postbaseline scores; within-subject area under the curve (AUC); and within-subject time to reach a prespecified value.

In the interpretation of results on PRO endpoints, statistical significance alone may not be meaningful. Therefore, the claims about treatment benefits should be accompanied by a well-justified responder definition and other data-presentation tools. To facilitate the interpretation of results from the analysis of PRO data, alternative approaches have been proposed, including the anchor-based and distribution-based approaches (see, e.g., Cappelleri et al. 2013; Marquis et al. 2004; McLeod et al. 2011). An anchor-based approach attempts to link the targeted concept that the PRO is intended to measure to an anchor measure or indicator that is interpretable itself or lends itself to interpretation. Thus, while the anchor may or may not be another PRO measure, it is required to meet at least two criteria: viz., be correlated with the targeted PRO, and be easy to interpret relative to the PRO of interest. Anchor-based methods include percentages based on thresholds. For example, when using incontinence diaries that also collect the number of incontinence episodes, the mean change in PRO scores corresponding to a 50% reduction in episodes may be used to define a responder. Similarly, when patients are blinded to treatment assignment, their assessment of change recorded at different times may be used to define a responder. Specifically, the difference in PRO scores corresponding to the change in ratings (better/same vs. worse) can serve to define a responder (FDA 2009).

Distribution-based approaches, often used as supportive tools, typically relate to the magnitude of a treatment effect, both at the individual and group levels (Alemayehu and Cappelleri 2012). Examples of distributed-based approaches for a group of patients include standard error of measurements (SEM), and cumulative distribution of response curves (FDA 2009). The US FDA encourages the use of the cumulative distribution function (CDF) of responses between treatment groups, including an application of the responder definition along the CDF curve at each level of response (FDA 2009).

Figure 4.2 illustrates a CDF plot in which the solid and dashed curves denote the distributions for the two treatment groups. Assuming negative change scores indicate improvement, for example, at a change score of –2 (i.e., a 2-point improvement), where higher scores represent worse condition, the difference in the corresponding percentage of subjects is Δ = 25%.

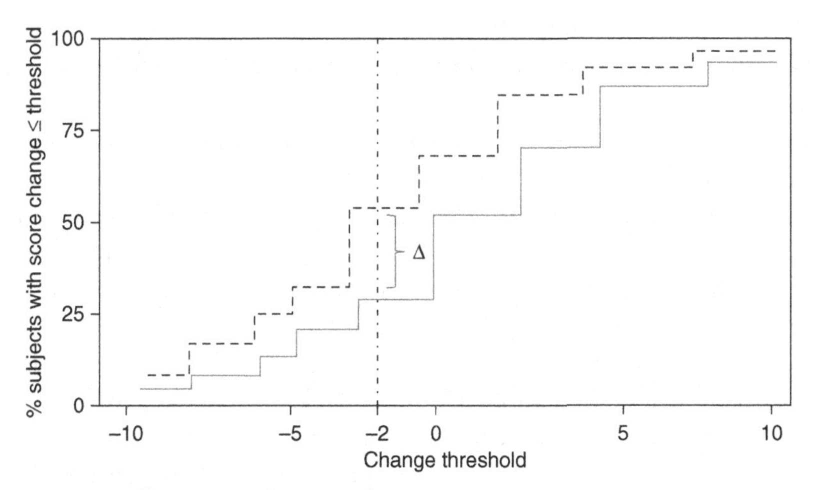

FIGURE 4.2 Illustration of a CDF Plot

When composite endpoints are constructed combining the scores from multiple items or domains, there should be clarity about the interpretation of the associated results, since the results may depend on the relative importance of the components and the corresponding effect sizes. When a composite endpoint shows favorable results, the component-wise results should be presented to indicate the relative contributions to the favorable result.

In certain situations, PRO instruments can be used to capture safety data, especially when it is deemed important to elicit the information from the patient perspective. In cancer trials, there have been ongoing efforts to streamline and harmonize the collection of safety data as a central PRO concept. This includes the concept proposed the FDA Office of Hematology and Oncology Products (OHOP) (Kluetz et al. 2016), and the National Cancer Institute's Patient-Reported Outcomes version of the Common Terminology Criteria for Adverse Events (PRO-CTCAE). The latter is especially considered a useful tool to standardize the assessment of symptomatic AEs from the patient perspective (NIH NCI 2019).

4.2.5 Concluding Remarks

PROs have attracted considerable attention from regulatory agencies, payers, and pharmaceutical companies. Traditional clinical trials, which rely upon observer-reported outcomes, often fail to take into account the patients' perspective and experience. As patients get more involved in clinical trials and in their own healthcare, they will seek to have greater voice and greater access to data from other patients on trials to make informed decisions about their treatment. Thus, collecting reliable data that reflect the patients' perspectives is a critical component of drug development.

From a regulatory perspective, evidence gathered using a well-defined and reliable PRO instrument in appropriately designed trials can be used to support labeling claim. However, development and validation of a PRO instrument requires strict regulatory and psychometric requirements, which involve demonstration of the instrument's ability to reliably measure the claimed concept in the patient population enrolled in the clinical trial. Another issue of concern, especially in oncology, is the reliability of PRO data from open-label studies. As a consequence, despite the growing focus on the importance of PRO data, there is some variation in the degree to which regulatory agencies view the acceptability of such evidence for label claims. For example, according to a recent study, compared to the US FDA, the EMA tends to be more likely to accept data from open-label studies and broad concepts such as health-related quality of life (Gnanasakthy et al. 2019).

One major barrier that limits the wider use of PROs by healthcare systems in general is the scarcity of best practices in the use of validated instruments, especially when the comparability of data collected from disparate sources is desired. One framework, mentioned earlier, is the Patient-Reported Outcomes Measurement Information System (PROMIS), which aims to enhance and standardize measurement of several selected PROs. While the PROMIS network is growing, and actively developing and validating PROs in several new domains, it is still far from getting acceptance by regulatory agencies.

4.3 ARTIFICIAL INTELLIGENCE AND MODERN ANALYTICS IN REGULATORY SETTINGS

4.3.1 Introduction

It is widely acknowledged that the digital revolution has considerable potential to transform medical research and drug development, as has been the case in other areas of human endeavors (Alemayehu and Berger 2016; Mayer-Schönberger et al. 2014). Smart algorithms and powerful computing resources are now available to process and analyze huge volumes of data collected from diverse sources and in a variety of forms to address important medical problems, especially those related to personalized and precision medicine (Panahiazar et al. 2014; Teli 2014). Unsurprisingly, the complexity, speed, and size of the data, as well as the new computing approaches, have presented unprecedented challenges and opportunities for drug development, regulatory reviews, and healthcare utilization and decision-making (Roski et al. 2014).

According to McCarthy (2007), artificial intelligence (AI) is "the science and engineering of creating intelligent machines," and may be viewed, in a broad sense, as the marriage of modern statistical predictive models with expert systems and machine-learning (ML) algorithms. AI has come a long way since its inception by Turing (Turing 1950), with a wide range of applications, including image recognition, speech detection, and robotics. A major factor in the success of AI in medical research is the advance made in the development of powerful predictive models (Emir et al. 2017). Figure 4.3 depicts the ML prediction paradigm, which involves an iterative

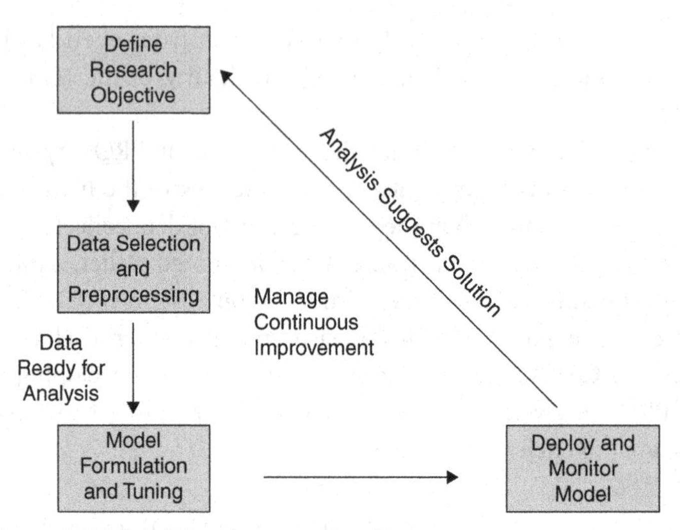

FIGURE 4.3 ML Model Development Paradigm

process of model development and validation, using training and test-data sets (Hastie et al. 2009; Shmueli 2010).

Interestingly, the methodological development in ML has been driven not just by statisticians and mathematicians, but also by researchers in other disciplines, including computer scientists and software engineers (Goodfellow et al. 2016). Classification and regression trees, including random forests (Breiman 2001a; 2001b), as well as penalized-regression methods (Hastie et al. 2009), are now in routine use in medical research. Other analytic tools include k-nearest neighbors (Dixon 1979), neural networks and deep learning (inspired by Rosenblatt (1958) and enhanced by Rumelhart et al. (1986)), and support vector machines (Vapnik 1995).

Deep learning models have especially been used in various applications in medical research. Notable architectures of such models include Convolutional Neural Networks (CNNs), restricted Boltzmann machines (RBMs) such as deep belief networks (DBNs), stacked Autoencoders, and recurrent neural networks (RNNs). The range of applications also includes bioinformatics (e.g., cancer diagnosis, gene classification, drug design, etc.), medical imaging (e.g., tissue classification and tumor detection), prediction of disease, and study of infectious disease epidemics (Ravi et al. 2017).

In this section we provide some potential use cases of AI in drug development, including approved examples of algorithms that have gone through FDA reviews. Since the use of real-world evidence in a regulatory setting is discussed elsewhere in this monograph, the focus in this section will be on specific applications of AI and ML tools.

4.3.2 AI in Drug Development

In the face of increasing costs of research and development (R&D), a major concern of the pharmaceutical industry is to explore ways of enhancing productivity and efficiency. Pharmaceutical companies are, therefore, attracted by the recent advancements in AI technology to transform the drug-development process, from early discovery through loss of exclusivity.

In the initial steps of drug development, ML algorithms can help in the identification of new or novel compounds with interesting biological activities. Modern predictive models permit incorporation of information from high-dimensional data, including genomics and relevant biochemical features (see, e.g., Wang et al. 2017). The approach can also be used for drug repurposing, in which an existing treatment option is considered to treat a new disease. As an example, in one instance an AI system involving neural networks was used to classify drugs into categories defined by transcriptional profiles (Aliper et al. 2016).

A promising area of application of AI and ML is prediction of the outcomes of drug-development programs to support go/no-go decisions, especially in the early phase, using preclinical or Phase I data, as well as other relevant data from the literature or available in the public domain. In a recent publication, Beinse et al. (2019) demonstrated the performance of an ML algorithm in predicting the time to FDA approval in oncology right after Phase I. Similarly, reliable prediction of toxicity in the preclinical phase may help to make informed decisions about the need to run subsequent clinical trials. As reported in Wu and Wang (2018), ML methods, such as deep learning, random forests, k-nearest neighbors, and support vector machines, have been applied to toxicity prediction, employing data not only from chemical structural descriptions, as is done customarily, but also genetic and other information.

A potential application of AI is in precision medicine, which requires the integration of data from diverse sources, including patient, drug, and environmental factors. Advanced machine learning models will enable use of the vast digital information to transform medical practice, by tailoring treatment of individual patients. While the application is still at the concept stage, there are efforts to accelerate use of the available AI tools and digital data to advance precision medicine (see, e.g., Kim et al. 2019).

AI has also applications in enhancing operational aspects of clinical trials, including site and patient selection, risk-based monitoring, and proactively assessing data-quality issues. For example, inclusion of patients in the trial may be based on reliable biomarkers that are identified using modern analytic tools. In one application, a novel AI platform has been implemented to monitor patient compliance (Bain et al. 2017).

4.3.3 Regulatory Experience with Machine Learning and Artificial Intelligence

Regulatory agencies have recognized the significance of AI and ML in providing new and important insights in the delivery of healthcare and are in the process of formulating relevant framework for the proper use of these technologies. A case in point is the recently proposed framework that the US FDA issued relating to AL/ML-based software as a medical device (FDA 2019b). The agency has also outlined good ML practices, as a total product lifecycle regulatory approach to continually improve the performance while limiting degradations (FDA 2019b).

In the EU the EMA has highlighted, among the strategic goals it formulated recently, the exploitation of the digital technology and artificial intelligence in decision-making (EMA 2018). As part of the scheme, the agency recommends, among others, the establishment of an AI laboratory and the building of capabilities in relevant areas, such as cognitive computing, that have applications in the regulatory system.

The US FDA has accepted use of certain AI algorithms for medical devices. Topol (2019) provided a list of at least fourteen approvals in 2017 and 2018 in several therapeutic areas. For example, in ophthalmology, FDA approved an autonomous AI system to detect diabetic retinopathy using data from a prospective trial conducted in primary-care settings compared to the historic gold standard (Abramoff et al. 2018). In cardiology, Apple received FDA approval for their electrocardiogram (ECG) algorithm used with the Apple Watch Series 4 and 5 to detect signs of arrhythmias for those older than 22 years (Victory 2018). However, it is not intended to provide a diagnosis (Buhr 2017; Fingas 2018). In pathology, QuantX was approved by the FDA as a platform that uses AI as an adjunct tool for assisting radiologists to analyze the breast ultrasound images of patients with soft tissue breast lesions (www.accessdata.fda.gov/cdrh_docs/reviews/DEN170022.pdf).

The standard practice for glucose monitoring in diabetic patients is the use of an invasive procedure. In September 2017 the FDA approved a continuous glucose monitoring system, in which the sensor continuously measures the glucose level every minute and can also provide graphics and summary statistics for glucose history through a handheld device (Bolinder et al. 2016).

Finally, signal detection is an important framework for identification of a risk for developing a drug adverse event after being exposed to it. vigiRank is a predictive model for emerging safety signals using the VigiBase (Caster et al. 2017). Ordinarily the disproportionality analysis is based on assessing disproportionality in pharmacovigilance data by observed-expected ratios (Zink et al. 2013). Caster et al. (2017) showed that vigiRank has outperform disproportionality analysis in real-world pharmacovigilance signal detection. Similarly, the European Medicines Agency developed a predictive signal-detection algorithm and applied to the EudraVigilance database that showed encouraging results (Pinheiro et al. 2018).

4.3.4 Concluding Remarks

With recent improvements in computer algorithms, many activities in our daily lives are increasingly relying on AI and ML applications. Unsurprisingly, regulatory bodies and pharmaceutical companies have begun to recognize the potential of the rapidly growing technology to enhance drug development and medical research. However, unlike in other industries, AI and ML appear to play very limited roles in the drug development and approval space. The recent approvals by FDA of limited algorithms in medical devices are examples of the degree of interest of the agency in the new technology.

With the skyrocketing cost of drug development, pharmaceutical companies are aggressively looking into the possibility of leveraging AI technology to improve productivity and efficiency. Advanced predictive models, coupled with rich databases, could be used to inform decision-making about drug discovery, continuation of development programs, or planning clinical-trial operations. In addition, there is considerable potential to advance the field of precision medicine, which depends on synthesizing vast digital information to tailor treatment to individual patients.

BIBLIOGRAPHY

Abramoff, M., Lavin, P. T., Birch, M. et al. (2018) Pivotal trial of an autonomous AI-based diagnostic system for detection of diabetic retinopathy in primary care offices. *NPJ Digital Medicine.* 1: 39.

Alemayehu, D., Berger, M. L. (2016) Big Data: Transforming drug development and health policy decision making. *Health Services and Outcomes Research Method.* 16: 92. https://doi.org/10.1007/s10742-016-0144-x.

Alemayehu, D., Cappelleri, J. C. (2012) Conceptual and analytical considerations toward the use of patient-reported outcomes in personalized medicine. *American Health & Drug Benefits.* 5(5): 310–317.

Alemayehu, D., Cappelleri, J. C. (2014) Patient-reported outcomes in personalized medicine. In: *Clinical and Statistical Considerations in Personalized Medicine.* Carini, C., Menon, S. M., Chang, M. editors. Boca Raton, FL: Chapman and Hall/CRC: 297–312.

Alemayehu, D., Mardekian, J. (2011) Infrastructure requirements for secondary data sources in comparative effectiveness research. *Journal of Managed Care & Specialty Pharmacy.* 17: S16–21.

Aliper, A., Plis, S., Artemov, A. et al. (2016) Deep learning applications for predicting pharmacological properties of drugs and drug repurposing using transcriptomic data. *Molecular Pharmaceutics.* 13 (7): 2524–2530.

Alphs, L., Mao, L., Lynn Starr, H., Benson, C. (2016) A pragmatic analysis comparing once-monthly paliperidone palmitate versus daily oral antipsychotic treatment in patients with schizophrenia. *Schizophrenia Research.* 170: 259–264.

Anglemyer A, Horvath H. T, Bero L. (2014) Healthcare outcomes assessed with observational study designs compared with those assessed in randomized trials. Cochrane Database of Systematic Reviews 2014, Issue 4. Art. No.: MR000034. DOI: 10.1002/14651858.MR000034.pub2.

Austin, P. C. (2007) The performance of different propensity score methods for estimating marginal odds ratios. *Statistics in Medicine.* 26: 3078–3094.

Austin, P. C. (2009a) Some methods of propensity-score matching had superior performance to others: Results of an empirical investigation and Monte Carlo simulations. *Biometrical Journal.* 51: 171–184.

Austin, P. C. (2009b) Type I error rates, coverage of confidence intervals, and variance estimation in propensity-score matched analyses. *International Journal of Biostatistics.* 5: Article 13. DOI: 10.2202/1557–4679.114.

Bain, E. E., Shafner, L., Walling, D. P., Othman, A. A., Chuang-Stein, C., Hinkle, J., Hanina, A. (2017) Use of a novel artificial intelligence platform on mobile devices to assess dosing compliance in a Phase 2 clinical trial in subjects with schizophrenia. *JMIR Mhealth and Uhealth.* 5: Article e18.

Bartlett, V. L., Dhruva, S. S., Shah, N. D., Ryan, P., Ross, J. S. (2019) Feasibility of using real-world data to replicate clinical trial evidence. *Journal of American Medical Association Network Open*. 2(10): e1912869. DOI: https://doi.org/10.1001/jamanetworkopen.2019.12869.

Basch, E., Dueck A. C. (2016) Patient reported outcome measurement in drug discovery: A tool to improve accuracy and completeness of efficacy and safety data. *Expert Opinion on Drug Discovery*. 11(8): 753–758.

Baumfeld Andre, E., Reynolds, R., Caubel, P., Azoulay, L., Dreyer, N. A. (2019) Trial designs using real-world data: The changing landscape of the regulatory approval process. *Pharmacoepidemiology and Drug Safety*. 1–12. https://doi. org/10.1002/pds.4932.

Beinse, G., Tellier, V., Charvet, V. et al. (2019) Prediction of drug approval after phase I clinical trials in oncology: RESOLVED2. *JCO Clinical Cancer Informatics*. 3: 1–10.

Benson, K, Hartz, A. J. (2000) A Comparison of Observational Studies and Randomized, Controlled Trials, New England Journal of Medicine, V. 342;1878 -1886, doi: 10.1056/NEJM200006223422506

Berger, M. L., Mamdani, M., Atkins, D. et al. (2009) Good research practices for comparative effectiveness research: Defining, reporting and interpreting nonrandomized studies of treatment effects using secondary data sources: The International Society for Pharmacoeconomics and Outcomes Research Good Research Practices for Retrospective Database Analysis Task Force Report – Part 1. *Value in Health*. 12: 1044–1052.

Berger, M. L, Martin, B. C., Husereau, D. et al. (2014) A questionnaire to assess the relevance and credibility of observational studies to inform health care decision making: An ISPOR-AMCP-NPC Good Practice Task Force Report. *Value in Health*. 17: 143–156.

Bolinder, J. Antuna, R., Geelhoed-Duijvestijn, P., et al. (2016) Novel glucose-sensing technology and hypoglycemia in type 1 diabetes: A multicentre, non-masked, randomised controlled trial. *The Lancet*. 388(10057): 2254–2263.

Bosco, J. L., Silliman, R. A., Thwin, S. S. et al. (2010) A most stubborn bias: No adjustment method fully resolves confounding by indication in observational studies. *Journal of Clinical Epidemiology*. 63: 64–74.

Brookhart, M. A., Wang, P. S., Solomon, D. H. et al. (2006) Evaluating short-term drug effects in claims databases using physician-specific prescribing preferences as an instrumental variable. *Epidemiology*. 17: 268–275.

Breiman, L. (2001a) Random forests. *Machine Learning*. 45: 5–32.

Breiman, L. (2001b) Statistical modeling: The two cultures (with comments and a rejoinder by the author). *Statistical Science*. 16: 199–231.

Buhr, S. (2017) FDA clears AliveCor's Kardiaband as the first medical device accessory for the Apple Watch. In TechCrunch https://techcrunch. com/2017/11/30/fda-clears-alivecors-kardiaband-as-the-first-medicaldevice-accessory-for-the-apple-watch/.

Cappelleri, J. C., Zou, K. H., Bushmakin, A. G., Alvir, J. M. J., Alemayehu, D., Symonds, T. (2013) *Patient-Reported Outcomes: Measurement, Implementation and Interpretation*. Boca Raton: Chapman & Hall/CRC Press (Taylor & Francis).

Carpenter, J. R., Kenward, M. G. (2013) *Multiple Imputation and Its Application*. New York: John Wiley & Sons.

Caster, O., Sandberg, L., Bergvall, T., Watson, S., Norén, G. (2017) vigiRank for statistical signal detection in pharmacovigilance: First results from prospective real-world use. *Pharmacoepidemiology and Drug Safety*. 26(8): 1006–1010. www.ncbi.nlm.nih.gov/pubmed/28653790.

Cella, D., Yount, S., Rothrock, N., Gershon, R., Cook, K., Reeve, B., Ader, D., Fries, J. F., Bruce, B., Rose, M. (2007) for the PROMIS Cooperative Group. The Patient-Reported Outcomes Measurement Information System (PROMIS): Progress of an NIH Roadmap cooperative group during its first two years. *Medical Care*. 45 (5 Suppl 1): S3–S11.

Collins, L. M., Lanza, S. T. (2009) *Latent Class and Latent Transition Analysis: With Applications in the Social, Behavioral, and Health Sciences*. Hoboken: John Wiley & Sons.

Cochran, W. G. (1968) The effectiveness of adjustment by subclassification in removing bias in observational studies. *Biometrics*. 24: 295–313.

Cooper, C., Booth, A., Varley-Campbell, J., Britten, N., & Garside, R. (2018). Defining the process to literature searching in systematic reviews: a literature review of guidance and supporting studies. BMC medical research methodology, 18(1), 85. https://doi.org/10.1186/s12874-018-0545-3

D'Agostino, R. B. (1998) Propensity score methods for bias reduction in the comparison of a treatment to a nonrandomized control group. *Statistics in Medicine*. 17: 2265–2281.

de Ayala, R. J. (2005) *The Theory and Practice of Item Response Theory*. New York: Guilford Press.

Deeks, J. J., Dinnes, J., D'Amico, R. et al. (2003) Evaluating non-randomised intervention studies. *Health Technology Assessment*. 7: iii-x, 1–173.

DeWalt, D. A., Rothrock, N., Yount, S., Stone, A. A. (2007) PROMIS Cooperative Group. Evaluation of item candidates: The PROMIS qualitative item review. *Medical Care*. 45: S12–S21.

Dixon, J. K. (1979) Pattern recognition with partly missing data. *IEEE Transactions on Systems, Man, and Cybernetics*. 9: 617–621.

Drummond, M. F., Torrance, G. W. (2005) *Methods for the Economic Evaluation of Health Care Programmes*. Oxford: Oxford University Press.

Emir, B., Gruben,D. C., Bhattacharyya, H. T., Reisman, A. L., Cabrera, J. (2017). *Predictive Modelling in HEOR. Statistical Topics in Health Economics and Outcomes Research.* (pp 69–82). New York, NY: CRC Press.

European Medicines Agency (2016) Appendix 2 to the guideline on the evaluation of anticancer medicinal products in man. The use of patient-reported outcome (PRO) measures in oncology studies. www.ema.europa.eu/en/documents/other/appendix-2-guideline-evaluation-anticancer-medicinal-products-man_en.pdf (accessed August 28, 2019).

European Medicines Agency (2018) EMA regulatory science to 2025. Strategic reflection. www.ema.europa.eu/en/documents/regulatory-procedural-guideline/ema-regulatory-science-2025-strategic-reflection_en.pdf.

Fairclough, D. L. (2010) *Design and Analysis of Quality of Life Studies in Clinical Trials.* 2nd ed. Boca Raton: Chapman & Hall/CRC.

Fingas, R. (2018) Apple Watch Series 4 EKG tech got FDA clearance less than 24 hours before reveal. In AppleInsider. https://appleinsider.com/ articles/18/09/18/apple-watch-series-4-ekg-tech-got-fda-clearance-less-than- 24-hours-before-reveal.

Fitzmaurice, G. M., Laird, N. M., Ware, J. H. (2011) *Applied Longitudinal Analysis.* 2nd ed. Hoboken: John Wiley & Sons.

Food and Drug Administration (2001) E10 choice of control group and related issues in clinical trials. (accessed December 27, 2019).

Food and Drug Administration (2009) Guidance for industry on patient-reported outcome measures: Use in medical product development to support labeling claims. *Federal Register.* 74(235): 65132–65133.

Food and Drug Administration (2013) Best practices for conducting and reporting pharmacoepidemiologic safety studies using electronic healthcare data. (Pharmacoepidemiologic Guidance). (accessed December 27, 2019).

Food and Drug Administration (2018a) Framework for the FDA's Real World Evidence Program. www.fda.gov/media/120060/download. (accessed December 29, 2019).

Food and Drug Administration (2018b) US FDA qualification letter. www.fda.gov/media/115635/download (accessed September 17, 2019).

Food and Drug Administration (2018c) Use of electronic health record data in clinical investigations guidance for industry, July 2018. Framework for FDA's real-world evidence program, December 2018. Submitting documents using real-world data and real-world evidence to FDA for drugs and biologics draft guidance for industry. May 2019. www.fda.gov/science-research/science-and-research-special-topics/real-world-evidence.

Food and Drug Administration (2019a) Press release palbociclib approved by FDA for treatment of male patients with HR+/HER2- breast cancer. www.targetedonc.com/news/palbociclib-approved-by-fda-for-treatment-of-male-patients-with-hrher2-breast-cancer. (accessed July 19, 2019).

Food and Drug Administration (2019b) Proposed regulatory framework for modifications to AI/ML based software as a medical device. www.fda.gov/medical-devices/software-medical-device-samd/artificial-intelligence-and-machine-learning-software-medical-device (accessed September 17, 2019).

Franklin J. M, Schneeweiss S. (2017) When and How Can Real World Data Analyses Substitute for Randomized Controlled Trials?. Clin Pharmacol Ther.102(6): 924–933. doi:10.1002/cpt.857

Fröbert, O., Lagerqvist, B., Olivecrona, G., Omerovic, E., Gudnason, T., Maeng, M., Aasa, M., Angerås, O., Calais, F., Danielewicz, M., Erlinge, D., Hellsten, L., Jensen, U., Johansson, A.C., Kåregren, A., Nilsson, J., Robertson, L., Sandhall, L., Sjögren, I., Östlund, O., Harnek, J., James, S. K. (2013) Thrombus aspiration during ST-segment elevation myocardial infarction. *New England Journal of Medicine*. 369: 1587–1597.

Gaffney, M., Mardekian, J. (2009) Propensity scores in the analysis of observational studies. *Biopharmaceutical Report.* (16)3: 90–97.

Gaudino, M., Di Franco, A., Rahouma, M., Tam, D.Y., Iannaccone, Deb, S., D'Ascenzo, F. , Abouarab, A.A., Girardi, L.N., Taggart, D.P., Fremes, S.E. (2018) Unmeasured Confounders in Observational Studies Comparing Bilateral Versus Single Internal Thoracic Artery for Coronary Artery Bypass Grafting: A MetaAnalysis, Journal of the American Heart Association, 7, e008010

Gnanasakthy, A., Barrett, A., Evans, E., D'Alessio, D., Romano, C. D. (2019) A review of patient-reported outcomes labeling for oncology drugs approved by the FDA and the EMA (2012–2016). *Value in Health*. 22(2): 203–209.

Gokbuget, N., Dombret, H., Bonifacio, M. et al. (2018) Blinatumomab for minimal residual disease in adults with B-cell precursor acute lymphoblastic leukemia. *Blood.* 131: 1522–1531.

Goodfellow, I., Bengio, Y., Courville, A. (2016) *Deep Learning*. Cambridge: MIT Press.

Hambleton, R. K., Swaminathan, H., Rogers, H. J. (1991) *Fundamentals of Item Response Theory*. Newbury Park: Sage Publications.

Hastie, T., Tibshirani, R., Friedman, J. (2009) *The Elements of Statistical Learning: Data Mining, Inference and Prediction*. 2nd ed. New York: Springer.

Hays, R. D., Morales, L. S., Reise, S. P. (2000) Item response theory and health outcomes measurement in the 21st century. *Medical Care*. 38(9, supplement II): II-28–II-42.

Heckman, J. J. (2005) The scientific model of causality. *Sociological Methodology*. 35: 1–97.

Hedeker, D., Gibbons, R. D. (2006) *Longitudinal Data Analysis*. Hoboken: John Wiley & Sons.

Hemkens, L. G., Contopoulos-Ioannidis, D. G., Ioannidis, J. P. A. (2016) Agreement of treatment effects for mortality from routinely collected data and subsequent randomized trials: meta-epidemiological survey, BMJ 2016;352:i493

Hernandez, A. F., Fleurence, R. L., Rothman, R. L. (2015) The ADAPTABLE trial and PCORnet: Shining light on a new research paradigm. *Annals of Internal Medicine*. 163(8): 635–636.

ICH Harmonised Tripartite Guidelines on Choice of Control Group and Related Issues in Clinical Trials (ICH-E10) July 20, 2000. (accessed March 17, 2017]. Available from: www.ich.org/fileadmin/Public_Web_Site/ICH_Products/Guidelines/Efficacy/E10/Step4/E10_Guideline.pdf.

Imbens, G. W. (2004) Nonparametric estimation of average treatment effects under exogeneity: A review. *Review of Economics and Statistics*. 86: 4–29.

Kim, Y. J., Kelley, B. P., Nasser, J. S., Chung, K. C. (2019) Implementing precision medicine and artificial intelligence in plastic surgery: Concepts and future prospects. *Plastic and Reconstructive Surgery Global Open*. 7(3), March 11: e2113. DOI: 10.1097/GOX.0000000000002113.

Kleinbaum, D. G., Sullivan, K. M., Barker, N. D. (2013) *ActiveEpi Companion Textbook: A Supplement for Use with the ActiveEpi CD-ROM*. 2nd ed. New York: Springer.

Kluetz, P. G., Slagle, A., Papadopoulos, E. et al. (2016) Focusing on core patient-reported outcomes in cancer clinical trials: Symptomatic adverse events, physical function, and disease-related symptoms. *Clinical Cancer Research*. 22: 1553–1558.

Little, R. J. A. (1993) Pattern-mixture models for multivariate incomplete data. *Journal of the American Statistical Association*. 88: 125–134.

Little, R. J. A., Rubin, D. B. (2002) *Statistical Analysis with Missing Data*. 2nd ed. Hoboken: John Wiley & Sons.

Little, R. J. A., Rubin, D. B. (2019) *Statistical Analysis with Missing Data*. 3rd ed. Hoboken, NJ: John Wiley & Sons.

Lunceford, J. K., Davidian, M. (2004) Stratification and weighting via the propensity score in estimation of causal treatment effects: A comparative study. *Statistics in Medicine*. 23: 2937–2960.

Madigan, D., Ryan, P. B., Schuemie, M. J. et al. (2013a) Evaluating the impact of database heterogeneity on observational study results. *American Journal of Epidemiology*. 15: 645–651.

Madigan, D., Schuemie, M. J., Ryan, P. (2013b) Empirical performance of the case–control method: Lessons for developing a risk identification and analysis system. *Drug Safety*. 36: 73–82.

Marquis, P., Chassany, O., Abetz, L. (2004) A comprehensive strategy for the interpretation of quality-of-life data based on existing methods. *Value in Health*. 7: 93–104.

Mayer-Schönberger, V., Cukier, K. (2014) *Big Data: A Revolution that Will Transform How We Live, Work and Think*. London: Eamon Dolan/Mariner Books.

McCarthy J. (2007). What is artificial intelligence? Available at: http://jmc.stanford.edu/articles/whatisai/whatisai.pdf (Accessed on August 14, 2020).

McClellan, M., McNeil, B. J., Newhouse, J. P. (1994) Does more intensive treatment of acute myocardial infarction in the elderly reduce mortality? Analysis using instrumental variables. *Journal of American Medical Association.* 272: 859–866.

McLeod, L. D., Coon, C. D., Martin, S. A. et al. (2011) Interpreting patient-reported outcome results: US FDA guidance and emerging methods. *Expert Review of Pharmacoeconomics & Outcomes Research.* 11: 163–169.

Mendell, J. R., Goemans, N., Lowes, L. P. et al. (2016) Longitudinal effect of eteplirsen versus historical control on ambulation in Duchenne muscular dystrophy. *Annals of Neurology.* 79: 257–271.

Newhouse, J. P., McClellan, M. (1998) Econometrics in outcomes research: The use of instrumental variables. *Annual Review of Public Health.* 19: 17–34.

NIH, National Cancer Institute (2019) Patient-Reported Outcomes version of the Common Terminology Criteria for Adverse Events (PRO-CTCAE™) https://healthcaredelivery.cancer.gov/pro-ctcae/ (accessed August 26, 2019).

O'Kelly, M., Ratitch, B. (2014) *Clinical Trials with Missing Data: A Guide for Practitioners.* Hoboken: John Wiley & Sons.

Panahiazar, M., Taslimitehrani, V., Jadhav, A., Pathak, J. (2014) Empowering personalized medicine with big data and semantic web technology: Promises, challenges, and use cases. *Proceedings of the IEEE International Conference on Big Data.* DOI: 10.1109/BigData.2014.7004307.

Patrick, D. L., Burke, L. B., Gwaltney, C. H., Kline Leidy N., Martin, M. L., Molsen, E., Ring, L. (2011a) Content validity – Establishing and reporting the evidence in newly developed patient reported outcomes (PRO) instruments for medical product evaluation: ISPOR PRO good research practices task force report: Part 1 – Eliciting concepts for a new PRO instrument. *Value in Health.* 14: 967–977.

Patrick, D. L., Burke, L. B., Gwaltney, C. H., Kline Leidy, N., Martin, M. L., Molsen, E., Ring, L. (2011b) Content validity – Establishing and reporting the evidence in newly developed patient reported outcomes (PRO) instruments for medical product evaluation: ISPOR PRO good research practices task force report: Part 2 – Assessing respondent understanding. *Value in Health.* 14: 978–988.

Pinheiro, L., Candore, G., Zaccaria, C., Slattery, J., Arlett, P. (2018) An algorithm to detect unexpected increases in frequency of reports of adverse events in EudraVigilance. *Pharmacoepidemiology and Drug Safety.* 27(1): 38–45. www.ncbi.nlm.nih.gov/pubmed/29143393.

Porter, J., Love, D., Costello, A. et al. (2015) All-payer claims database development manual: Establishing a foundation for health care transparency and informed decision making. APCD Council and West Health Policy Center. Available at: www.apcdcouncil.org/manual. (accessed July 1, 2016).

Psaty, B. M., Siscovick, D. S. (2010) Minimizing bias due to confounding by indication in comparative effectiveness research: The importance of restriction. *Journal of American Medical Association.* 304: 897–898.

Public Law No: 114-255 (December 13, 2016). www.congress.gov/bill/114th-congress/house-bill/34/.

Robins, J. M., Hernan, M. A., Brumback, B. (2000) Marginal structural models and causal inference in epidemiology. *Epidemiology.* 11: 550–560.

Rosenbaum, P. R., Rubin, D. B. (1983) The central role of the propensity score in observational studies for causal effects. *Biometrika.* 70: 41–55.

Roski, J., Bo-Linn, G. W., Andrews, T. (2014) Creating value in health care through big data: Opportunities and policy implications. *Health Affairs. (Project Hope).* 33(7): 1115–1122. www.ncbi.nlm.nih.gov/pubmed/25006136.

Ravi, D., Wong, W., Deligianni, F. et al. (2017) Deep learning for health informatics. *IEEE Journal of Biomedical and Health Informatics.* 21: 4–21.

Rosenblatt, F. (1958) The perceptron: A probabilistic model for information storage and organization in the brain. *Psychological Review.* 65: 386–408.

Rumelhart, D. E., Hinton, G. E., Williams, R. J. (1986) Learning representations by back-propagating errors. *Nature.* 323: 533–536.

Schneeweiss, S., Rassen, J. A., Glynn, R. J. et al. (2009) High-dimensional propensity score adjustment in studies of treatment effects using health care claims data. *Epidemiology.* 20: 512–522.

Schneeweiss, S., Setoguchi, S., Brookhart, A. et al. (2007) Risk of death associated with the use of conventional versus atypical antipsychotic drugs among elderly patients. *Canadian Medical Association Journal.* 176: 627–632.

Setoguchi, S., Schneeweiss, S., Brookhart, M. A. et al. (2008) Evaluating uses of data mining techniques in propensity score estimation: A simulation study. *Pharmacoepidemiology and Drug Safety.* 17: 546–555.

Sherman, R. E., Anderson, S. A., Dal Pan, G. J. et al. (2016) Real-world evidence - what is it and what can it tell us? *New England Journal of Medicine.* 375: 2293–2297.

Shmueli, G. (2010) To explain or to predict? *Statistical Science.* 25: 289–310.

Singer, J. D., Willett, J. B. (2003) *Applied Longitudinal Data Analysis: Modeling Change and Event Occurrence.* New York: Oxford University Press.

Stukel, T. A. Fisher, E. S., Wennberg, D. E. et al. (2007) Analysis of observational studies in the presence of treatment selection bias. *Journal of American Medical Association.* 297: 278–285.

Sturmer, T., Joshi, M., Glynn, R. J. et al. (2006) A review of the application of propensity score methods yielded increasing use, advantages in specific settings, but not substantially different estimates compared with conventional multivariable methods. *Journal of Clinical Epidemiology*. 59: 437–447.

Sutter, S. (2016) Real-world evidence may find a home on breakthrough pathway. *Pink Sheet* 78/No. 26, June 27, 2016. www.focr.org/news/pink-sheet-real-world-evidence-may-find-home-breakthrough-pathway (accessed May 10, 2017).

Teli, N. (2014) Big Data: A catalyst for personalized medicine. http://healthcare-executive-insight.advanceweb.com/Features/Articles/Big-Data-A-Catalyst-for-Personalized-Medicine.aspx.

Tibshirani, R. (1996) Regression shrinkage and selection via the lasso. *Journal of the Royal Statistical Society. Series B Methodological.* 58: 267–288.

Topol, E. (2019) High-performance medicine: The convergence of human and artificial intelligence. *Nature Medicine*. 25, January: 44–56.

Turing, A. M. (1950) Computing machinery and intelligence. *Mind*. 59: 433–460.

Vapnik, V. (1995) *The Nature of Statistical Learning Theory*. New York: Springer.

Victory, J. (2018) What did journalists overlook about the Apple Watch 'heart monitor' feature? In HealthNewsReview. www.healthnewsreview. org/2018/09/what-did-journalists-overlook-about-the-apple-watch-heartmonitor-feature/.

von Elm, E., Altman, D. G., Egger, M., Pocock. S. J.,, Gøtzsche, S. J., Vandenbroucke, J. P, for the STROBE Initiative (2008) The Strengthening the Reporting of Observational Studies in Epidemiology (STROBE) statement: Guidelines for reporting observational studies. *Journal of Clinical Epidemiology*. 61: 344–349.

Wang, Q. Feng, Y., Huang, J., Wang, Q., Feng, Y., Huang, J., Wang, T., Cheng, G. (2017) A novel framework for the identification of drug target proteins: Combining stacked auto-encoders with a biased support vector machine. *PLoS Medicine*. 12: Article e0176486.

Waning, B., Montagne, M. (2001) *Pharmacoepidemiology Principles and Practice*. New York: McGraw Hill.

Wu, Y., Wang, G. (2018) Machine learning based toxicity prediction: From chemical structural description to transcriptome analysis. *International Journal of Molecular Sciences*. 19(8), August 10: 2358. DOI: 10.3390/ijms19082358.

Zagadailov, E., Fine, M., Shields, A.(2013) Patient-reported outcomes are changing the landscape in oncology care: Challenges and opportunities for payers. *American Health & Drug Benefits*. 6(5): 264.

Zink, R. C., Huang, Q., Zhang, L. Y., Bao, W. J. (2013) Statistical and graphical approaches for disproportionality analysis of spontaneously-reported adverse events in pharmacovigilance. *Chinese Journal of Natural Medicines*. 11: 314–320.

Zou, H., Hastie, T. (2005) Regularization and variable selection via the elastic net. *Journal of the Royal Statistical Society. Series B (Statistical Methodology)*. 67: 301–320.

Index

Note: Page numbers in *italics* indicate *figures* and in **bold** indicate tables on the corresponding pages.

Printed in the United States
By Bookmasters